PARENTHOOD
LOST

PARENTHOOD
LOST

HEALING THE PAIN
AFTER MISCARRIAGE,
STILLBIRTH,
AND INFANT DEATH

WRITTEN AND EDITED BY
MICHAEL R. BERMAN, M.D.

FOREWORD BY SHERWIN B. NULAND

Bergin & Garvey
Westport, Connecticut • London

Library of Congress Cataloging-in-Publication Data

Parenthood lost : healing the pain after miscarriage, stillbirth, and infant death / written and edited by Michael R. Berman ; foreword by Sherwin B. Nuland.
    p. cm.
    Includes bibliographical references and index.
    ISBN: 9780313360930
      1. Grief. 2. Bereavement—Psychological aspects. 3. Infants—Death—
Psychological aspects. 4. Fetal death—Psychological aspects. 5. Stillbirth—
Psychological aspects. 6. Miscarriage—Psychological aspects. 7. Loss
(Psychology) I. Berman, Michael R.
    BF575.G7P366 2001
    155.9'37'085—dc21   00–029257

British Library Cataloguing in Publication Data is available.

Library of Congress Catalog Card Number: 00–029257
ISBN: 0–89789–614–9

First published in 2001

Bergin & Garvey, 88 Post Road West, Westport, CT 06881
An imprint of Greenwood Publishing Group, Inc.
www.greenwood.com

Printed in the United States of America

The paper used in this book complies with the
Permanent Paper Standard issued by the National
Information Standards Organization (Z39.48–1984).

10 9 8 7 6 5 4 3 2

Copyright Acknowledgments

The author and publisher gratefully acknowledge permission for use of the following material:

Excerpts from L. Väisänen, Family grief and recovery process when a baby dies, *Acta Universitatis Ouluensis D Medica 398* (1996), Oulu University Press, Oulu, Finland.

Windows

Gather
every morsel
of hope,
precious gift,
and open your eyes
to its wonder;
common images
earthly sights
hourly routines
that maintain
the equilibrium
of why and how
you live
and lived.
Delight
in what are your joys
and then
for just a brief moment
let them close
to the darkness
and paint
upon the canvas
of your soul
portraits
of secret longings
that come alive
in these minutes
of solitude
called dreaming,
art forms to dance
from the palette
as you revel in
this secret world
of unspoiled vision
and immortal promise.

CONTENTS

CONTENTS

PART III   REASONS FOR THE MOST COMMON PERINATAL LOSSES

CONTENTS

DEDICATION

This book has materially developed over a period of years; the content and thoughts have been gleaned over my professional lifetime. Its inspiration and thus its being has come from my *patients*, who were thrust into the tumult of sorrow when their child died. I wish this book were not needed, but humankind's history dictates otherwise. I therefore first dedicate this book to my *patients* and to all *families*, worldwide, who have endured these *unspeakable* losses.

My love for poetry was nurtured by my high school English teacher, Donald Fenton Hamingson, who died in 1998, at the age of sixty-nine. Donald Hamingson was an extraordinary individual and a role model for every one of his students. When I last saw him in 1993, he was still immersed in teaching the wonders and beauty of, and the reason for, poetry. It is my honor to recognize his effect on my life in this dedication.

Deepest expressions of gratitude must go to my wife, Nancy, and our daughters, Stephanie and Annie, who have so genuously understood and critiqued the writing of this book. I would also like to acknowledge my colleagues and mentors at the Yale University School of Medicine—Martin E. Gordon, M.D., Clinical Professor of Medicine; Sherwin B. Nuland, M.D., Clinical Professor of Surgery; Frederick Naftolin, M.D., D.Phil., Professor and Chairman, Department of Obstetrics and Gynecology; and Richard Seltzer, M.D., Clinical Professor of Surgery—for their support and encouragement during this process; my students, who have provided constant intellectual stimulation and feedback; my partners in medical practice at County Obstetrics and Gynecology Group; and my editor, Jane Garry, who approached me with the idea of this book, and without whose support this publication might not have been a reality.

FOREWORD

SHERWIN B. NULAND

The physicians of the Hippocratic era called medicine The Art, because they knew that the care of their fellows was an act of creativity. Even as they sought to identify signs, physical findings and other objective evidence of disease that all could agree upon, they also recognized that each patient and his or her physician form a bond that is unique unto itself. That bond is the foundation upon which healing takes place.

The bond's formation and maintenance is the fundamental aspect of The Art, no less a creative act than is healing itself. It has little to do with science, and a great deal to do with the human need to be understood. It goes beyond the notion of mere empathy and sometimes comes very near to being a kind of love. There are doctors whose ability to respond to the emotional needs of patients is so profound that wonder becomes a paramount factor in the way they are viewed by their colleagues. We are in awe of their ability to heal, even when their ability to cure is no greater than our own. Of the various ways in which The Art makes itself manifest, this may be the greatest of all. For cure is not always possible.

It is when we cannot cure that the bond of patient with doctor reaches its ultimate challenge, straining to bring acceptance and consolation to ease the days of those who cannot be relieved of their sickness, and also of those who love them. When the struggle is ended without cure, those who are left behind are not to be forgotten.

And so, there are poets among us. The physician who nurtures the rhythms and streamings of life is no less a poet than the literary craftsman who nurtures the rhythms and streamings of language. Both sense the harmonies of nature, and are part of them; both sense the harmonies of nature, and heal by leading others to their restorative wellsprings.

Such a poet is Dr. Michael Berman; he is of one and the other sort at the same time. Michael Berman's literary gifts draw inspiration from the depths of his heart, which is the heart of a skilled and devoted physician. His is the creativity of which poets like Homer first sung, and his is the creativity of which Hippocrates knew. His is the creativity that gives us the art and The Art.

A single example will suffice. In his training, Dr. Berman was taught by well-meaning mentors that parents must be protected from the "shock" of seeing their stillborn child who had succumbed to an outwardly visible birth defect. But once freed of the acquired carapace that so many of his colleagues so comfortably wore, he realized that love is far more healing than is protectiveness. He began to let mothers, and fathers too, hold their dead child, and he allowed the creation of the memories of those moments to become a continuity with the enduring love that had begun to develop as the embryo grew into a child. And then he wrote elegiac poetry about what had been experienced, and he encouraged the bereaved parents to do the same, as well as to express their fellings in prose. In this way, he learned to heal as he had never been taught.

> I know I cannot hold you for long,
> capturing you for my world.
> But, rest gently with me,
> if only for a moment,
> that I may treasure the memory
> and the beauty of the gift that you are.

This is the book that Michael Berman has written to tell the rest of us of his journey, and of the journeys taken by the many grieving parents to whom his poetry, his care and his gentle touch have been the balm that soothed the pain of their most difficult hours.

Love suffices, but healing of the bereaved is helped also by insight, and Dr. Berman has seen to it that this book is endowed with the perspectives of experienced nurses, social workers and physicians who comfort families when they are faced with such tragedy. And he recognizes that even clinical and scientific medical information is essential if parents are to come to terms with their losses, and with the inevitability of some of the circumstances that give rise to them. He has assembled a group of experts to explain the biological aspects of the most common reasons for perinatal losses, and they have done so in a lucid, accessible manner.

Many people will read this valuable book, and I hope large numbers of physicians will be among them. In this day of distancing, clinical detachment and biomedical therapeutics, our profession needs guides to lead us back to the essential humanity with which we should practice our Art. There can be no better guide than a man who, faced with the anguish of a distraught mother and a father, can bring them the consolation and the hope that his poetry expresses:

> There is triumph to taste,
> love to embrace;
> havens of hope to inhabit.

INTRODUCTION

Countless mothers and fathers and those close to them silently grieve, with little resolution, over the loss of their pregnancies, newborns, and children. Seeking release from their sorrow, they cry and yearn for solace and hope, many times for years following their loss; their cries are but a muted weeping of despair as a child so longed for is not born, or is not born alive, or cannot be conceived. Pained by these losses, they see their lives as devoid of hope. Yet they prevail, for within each of us is a timeless, enduring spark of divine *hope*, a uniquely human greatness that permits us to challenge adversity and courageously face the unexplainable suffering of our souls and bodies. To realize the existence of this divine hope is a most cherished purpose, for with it our lives have promise and reason.

Infertility, pregnancy loss, and neonatal illness and subsequent death are among the most painful losses we can experience, for they deny us a family and leave sightless our vision for immortality through generations of the future. Moreover, a child not born is denied the delight of reveling in the simple beauty and endless wonder of this divine hope.

Early in my obstetrical training during the 1970s, I was exposed to the trauma of fetal demise. I was taught by respected and caring mentors that if a baby was stillborn or born with a serious, "unsightly" birth defect, the physician should attempt to protect the parents from the "shock" of seeing their dead child by covering it with a blanket, quickly removing it from the delivery area, and sending the body to the morgue to be buried in an un-marked grave. It was *thought* that this was helping the parents. We were unaware of the necessity of allowing them to bond, grieve, and have closure. Then, one delivery changed my views. A patient of mine delivered a preterm baby, stillborn, with anencephaly. Anencephaly is a condition where there is incomplete development of the fetal cranium and forebrain. It is not com-patible with life. I was familiar with this condition and felt it might be too devastating for the parents to see, much less to hold, their child. However, as I spent time with them during the labor, I realized it was going to be very important for them to do just that: hold, kiss, hug, and form a bond with their son. When he was born, I covered the top of his head with a hat and placed him on his mother's abdomen. She held him as if he were alive, related how beautiful he was and how much she loved him. She did not *see* any birth defects; she saw only her child. This experience affected my management of the stillborn forever.

Recently, a patient of mine had a twin demise at 24 weeks into her pregnancy. She had had difficulty conceiving, and this was her first pregnancy. Her twins shared a common circulation and developed very early problems with this "twin to twin" transfusion syndrome. She received "high tech," state-of-the-art care at our hospital's maternal special care–high risk pregnancy unit, weekly ultrasound examinations, and therapeutic amniocentesis. She phoned me at 9 P.M. the day following her last amniocentesis and said that she had not felt the babies move. I met her at the hospital and confirmed the worst. Her sons had died. Immediately her reaction was "Oh, my God, this cannot be . . . my life will never be the same . . . how can I go on? Take the babies now . . . don't make me go through labor . . . don't send me home." With convulsive tremors, she wailed in despair. Her husband gave her much comfort. I cried with her. A nurse from the labor floor (who coincidentally was the codirector of our perinatal bereavement program) and I spent hours counseling her and her husband. I explained what I felt was the best for her medically and emotionally: for them to go home that night, together; cry; gather strength; and plan for the induction of labor and delivery the next day. The patient and her husband agreed, and the next day she delivered her twin sons. She held them for hours. Afterward, although filled with sorrow, she and her husband seemed at peace. She talked about her sons, clutched their memento box with their sons' pictures, and talked about their funeral and memorial service plans. At the memorial service, prayers were said and poems were read. She planted morning glory seeds at the graveside. Closure was accomplished. I do not think I have ever seen a patient demonstrate such extremes in attitudes and emotions as the reality and circumstances of the day evolved, and I attribute this to the counseling she received and the way her children's deaths were approached.

In the last few years, awareness, compassion, intervention, and counseling have become the paradigm for the management of perinatal demise, yet even in the 1990s concern lingers that such mourning for a pregnancy loss is not fully accepted. ("There are no prayers for the matter of miscarriage, nor do we feel there should be."[1]) It is my hope that this book, rich with poems, stories, and insights into the impact of lost parenthood, will increase the awareness of and sensitivity to those who desperately need to assuage their profound sorrow; a sorrow of the ages, felt daily, worldwide, as we enter the new millennium.

Like strands of DNA, the very essence of life itself, the mourning of the demised unborn or newly born has traveled spiraled peaks and valleys.

My professional career has involved a striving to bring comfort and healing to children, born and yet to be born, and to mothers through their years of childbearing and beyond; it has been the cause in my life. I have been uplifted by the triumphs of birth and healing and depressed by the failures. Yet I have always tried to look beyond the failures in search of the triumphs. *Parenthood Lost: Healing the Pain after Miscarriage, Stillbirth, and Infant Death* is a journey and a journal of my feelings as an obstetrician. Here the reader will find uninhibited expressions of my emotions and of the mystical spirit of my participation in the processes of birth, of life, and of death, as well as testimony to optimism I have shared with my patients and that they have displayed through the years.

The stories of pregnancy and losses of children are recalled from my earliest contact with patients; some are written by my patients themselves; and others come from correspondence with parents I have never met. To preserve anonymity of the patient-contributors, I have omitted or changed identifications.

I have also included poems that I have written for children, mothers, fathers, and friends, with many of whom I have shared a part of their lives, or they, a part of mine. I have given or sent many of these poems to them or their families and, when appropriate, have recited them as eulogies at funerals and memorial services. The poems are original, unless otherwise noted, and have been written during my years as a practicing obstetrician. I have written notes as brief summaries and explanations of the inspirations for many of the poems. Others are simply defined by their title.

I have also included thoughts, poems, stories, and prayers from other caregivers who have tried to reach out to their patients and families.

The last part of the book, which gives the most common reasons for stillbirth and infant mortality, was written by practicing physicians.

.

PART I
POETRY

POETRY: COMFORTING THROUGH TIME

Though our spirits may fade and our viscera bleed,
we are enabled by the agents of our humanity
empowered by ancestral song and promise.

A child is not expected to die before his or her parents. The natural processes of birth, life, and death should follow in an orderly and rational sequence through one's lifetime. Any death other than one from *old age*, after a *rich* and fulfilling life, is premature. When parents see their child die, or carry the burden of an unborn child's demise, they live with this disruption of natural order forever. The value placed on the unborn and newly born has differed through generations and periods in human history, yet as value systems and moral codes evolved, in spite of rhetoric and practices of populations with regard to infanticide and population control, the profundity of a parent's grief has remained incontrovertible through the ages. There has not been, nor is there now, one common and standardized way to manage the recovery from such grief, for its shadow has been, and will be, indelibly imprinted in the minds and souls of these parents. Yet *forms* of expression implicit in symbolic language—poetry and verse, song, prayer and ritual—have served a role in all cultures and societies in dispelling the tears and fostering the healing from death and human loss.[1] Adult funeral services can talk of the *accomplishments* of the deceased, and describe joys and loves and relationships, through eulogies and memories. Yet when a newborn or young child dies or a child is not born alive, there is no personal history, seldom a long-standing relationship, few accomplishments, and barely a discernible personality to recount. However, a bond between mother and father and child or expected child exists and must be recognized. Death tears this apart. The issues of mourning, of lost promises, of sadness, and, above all, of maintaining *faith* must be addressed.

Why poetry? What forces implicit in its form and function move us and arouse our innermost yearnings and emotions? Why is the poetry of death a source of enduring inspiration and hope?

Poetry gives the patient a voice for his or her suffering. It may not alter the activity of the disease, but in merely providing a voice it comforts the patient in ways that no medication can.[2]

Poetry is a companion through dark times . . . a voice that makes it clear that you are not alone.[3]

Art [poetry], is human intelligence playing over the natural scene, ingeniously affecting it toward the fulfillment of human purpose.[4]

The Poet's gift . . . awakens in a special way the emotions of those who feel wordless in the face of loss.[5]

By making us stop for a moment, poetry gives us an opportunity to think about ourselves as human beings on this planet and what we mean to each other.[6]

Comfort may be achieved through the transfer of the poet's feelings into the reader's or listener's mind. Poetry transports the reader from the distractions and influences of the outside world, inward to the internal rhythms and solace of the personal soul. The poet becomes a healer, and his poetry, his staff. Through verse and meter, free of inhibition and full of expression, the poet may articulate a sensitivity and empathy and provoke introspection and inner peace. A poem is transformed into a message of hope. There is wonderment and magic in the words of a poem. Each word is selected for its individual meaning within the context of the entire poem. A few properly selected words can move the reader to tears and awaken the primal emotions of joy, despair, and *hope*. A poet should evoke emotion through his work and write as if each poem is his last work.[7]

The language of poetry, within the broader context of its "parent body" (literature), has always had as its great themes love, loss, and death.[8] The inclusion of *hope* among these thematic elements is worthwhile, if not essential, for (as humans) we *have* the capacity to bring hope to a despair that is uniquely created by our humanity and our human conditions.

Bereavement over the loss of a pregnancy, newborn, or young child is as old as mankind. My search into the origins of the use of a poem's graceful yet penetrating ability to soothe, into the essence of what its fragile words can create through symbolism, metaphor, and rhythm,[9] has led me to the portal of precivilization, more than 35,000 years ago. Here began this understanding of the primitive, even primal, urges for consolation for grieving parents.

In the dust where we have buried the silent races.[10]

Human culture emerged between 35,000 and 32,000 years ago (BP, before the present), in an archaeological period known as the upper Paleolithic or late Ice Age. This was marked by the biological evolution of modern human beings, subspecies *Homo sapiens sapiens*. With this evolution into modernity from the Mousterian culture[11] and from our ancestral Neanderthal species, *Homo sapiens neanderthalensis* (100,000 to 35,000 years BP) came a "cultural explosion" marked by "symbolic behavior and language and the capacity to imagine."[12] It is of interest to note that 80,000–50,000 BP there is archaeological evidence of "purposeful and ritualized" burials. Such activity demonstrates that the Neanderthal Mousterians were able to conceptualize death in such a way as to establish conventions to deal with its disruptive forces and externalize the emotional responses to it.[13] This "cultural coding"[14] is not unlike what has been said of poetry today. With poetry "the world of external reality recedes and the world of instinct, the effective emotional linkage behind the words, rises to the view and becomes the world of reality."[15] Primitive humans needed to survive the perils of their environment before they could learn to "live beautifully or create beautiful things."[16] However, a "primitive imagination flourished in the midst of this peril,"[17] and out of their concern for their physical suffering and disability, these primitive humans developed religious rites that focused upon the origins of their disease and pain. Their sickbed became their cradle of religious myths and superstitions. The fear of death invoked many of these rituals and burial customs in order to repel the spirits of the deceased.[18] Yet from such thought also developed behavior, rituals, and symbols to safeguard the females from the perils of childbirth and to memorialize their dead children.[19] One might consider that these death rituals of the Mousterians were the precursors of our contemporary poetry and prayers of grieving, although no written record exists that could prove this hypothesis.

Remains of a Neanderthal child were found in Siberia. The grave was surrounded by goat horns, deliberately placed in a symbolic pattern which demonstrated a very early expression of "animistic beliefs" that nature is personal and filled with the spirits which behave like human beings.[20]

Caves at Shanidar, in northeastern Iraq, were a rich source of Neanderthal excavations. This region of the world is considered by some to be the cradle of mankind, and evidence of purposeful burials, including the presence of small, brightly colored wildflowers, was found there. The remains of the Shanidar Man were found on a bed of woven, pinelike branches. Within the soil was pollen from several nonindigenous flowers, such as grape hyacinth, hollyhock, and yellow flowering groundsel. This has been "poetically" interpreted as evidence of the capacity for "human feelings" in prehuman species. The inhabitants of Shanidar buried their dead among nature's beauty after searching "the mountainside in the mournful task of collecting flowers.[21] One might imagine the recitation of a psalm or song, prayer or poem, in the manner we inter our loved ones today, in the death rituals of the Neanderthals as they buried their dead children amid the natural beauty of wildflowers.

This culture of the evolving *Homo sapiens sapiens* brought with it the cerebral attributes of "knowledge, belief, art, morals, custom and . . . other capabilities and habits acquired by man as a member of society."[22] A system of values developed along with the establishment of a moral code, and the value placed on *fertility* and *birth* in this period was among the highest. This is well documented by the abundant discoveries of fertility rituals and symbols displayed in cave drawings and portable art (pottery, stones, etc.). Birth, life, fertility, and transformation into death (regeneration), akin to the cycles of nature, predominate in Paleolithic and Neolithic images and are particularly strong themes in the image of the goddess and the symbolism contained within her language.[23] Richly painted artifacts emblazoned with depictions of life, in a wonderment of color and images, have been found. The goddess in all her manifestations was a symbol of the unity of all life in nature.[24] This makes us believe that the loss of a child, whether in utero or shortly after birth, was a great loss and evoked a grief response and a need that are evident through modernity. The enduring concepts of fertility, sterility, and "the fragility of life" are rooted in these Neolithic agricultural populations.[25] The egg, symbolic of birth and rebirth, was among the most ubiquitous symbols during this era. Its form abounds on vases and cave paintings of prehistoric periods.[26]

Discovery of wind instruments in southern France that were made some 32,000 years ago and the finding of small objects with parallel markings were early evidences of rhythmic arrangements and interval scales (Chatelperronian culture, 35,000–30,000 BP). Furthermore, recurrent patterns and structures of the Magdalenian culture (18,000–11,000 BP) show complex conceptualizations consistent with oral communication and development.[27] From this we might infer that symbolic representations recorded as a primitive language, along with the use of rhythm and music, may be considered ancestral to the emotional responses inherent in what we today consider poetry.

The Chinchorro people of Chile lived from 7000 B.C. to 5000 B.C. They revered their dead, particularly their children and their stillborn, and they put special effort into funerary rites and preservation by mummification. The process of such mummification is beyond the scope of our discussion, but the Chinchorros' commitment to this process was evident by their turning the simple body of a dead child into a complex work of art.[28] Generally, artificial mummification of dead children and fetuses was rare, for many primitive cultures did not consider them full members of society, yet it is evident this was not true for the Chinchorros. They had no written language, and an accurate account of their rituals is not possible. The mummification process was intended to preserve the dead indefinitely, for an "afterlife and ancestral worship."[29] Chinchorro mummies were buried with food and implements for the afterlife. The effort expended in this process of mummification leads one to believe that great value was placed on the lives, and therefore on the deaths, of these fetuses and children.[30]

The development of written language documented the rites and rituals connected with the death of a child. Much has been written and studied of the Egyptian's funerary practices of mummification. Their belief in life after death defined different spheres of a postmortem existence. Their spiritual being flourished after death.

Early in their civilization, the Egyptians planted their dead adults and children beneath the desert sand. When they were exhumed, intentionally or by wild animals, their bodies were discovered in a state of *natural* mummification, desiccated by the sun before they had begun to decompose. *Artificial* mummification is a purposeful desiccating process. The Egyptians utilized oils and wrapped the bodies to provide clothing. Funerary texts describing the relationships between the decreased and the gods were recited during the embalming and entombing. Such a text, a collection of magic spells and formulas, hymns and prayers, was written on papyrus, bound together, and collectively called *The Egyptian Book of the Dead*. It was thought that recitation of this text at time of death and entombing assured glorification in an afterlife. The book began to appear in Egyptian tombs around 1600 B.C. The text, intended to be spoken by the deceased during his or her journey into the underworld, was to enable the deceased to overcome obstacles in the afterlife. One pertinent allusion in the *Egyptian Book of the Dead* is to Hathor, the goddess of joy, motherhood, and love. She is called the "protectress of pregnant women," a midwife, a fertility goddess, and the patron of all women. She welcomes the deceased to the underworld, dispensing water to the souls of the dead from the branches of a sycamore and offering them food. "Hathor was also represented as a cow suckling the soul of the dead, thus giving them sustenance during their mummification, their journey to the judgement hall, and the weighing of their soul."[31] In later periods, dead women identified themselves with Hathor.

To better understand the use of poetics in the *Egyptian Book of the Dead*, I cite the following, which was recited to secure the affection of men, gods, and the spirit-souls for the deceased.

O my father Osiris, thou hast done for me that which thy father Ra did for thee. Let me abide upon the earth permanently. Let me keep possession of my throne. Let my heir be strong. Let my tomb, and my friends who are upon the earth, flourish. Let my enemies be given over to destruction, and to the shackles of the goddess Serq. I am thy son. Ra is my father. On me likewise thou hast conferred life, strength, and health. Horus is established upon my tomb. Grant thou that the days of my life may come unto worship and honour.[32]

The ancient Greeks and Romans held diverse and sometimes conflicting attitudes with regard to the worth of a child or a fetus. This is well documented, for their cultures were rich in literature and, in particular, poetics. Pregnant women in ancient Rome made a sacrifice of flowers to the goddess Juno, who was thought to have the power to prevent miscarriages.[33]

Yet the paradox of *infanticide* or "*exposure*" existed, not only for "defective" newborns but also for healthy ones. Infanticide, an old and almost universal custom, was commonly practiced in imperial Rome for reasons of poverty, vanity, malformations, population control, and other less defined social reasons. Many newborns—mostly female—were abandoned in the streets and left to perish or be sold as slaves or prostitutes.[34] It was felt by some that humanity was not conferred at birth. A higher value was placed on an ability to contribute than on just being human,[35] and failure to contribute rendered a human being "worthless." Children, according to the Greek philosopher Aristotle, were considered natural slaves of limited potential.[36] Plato and Aristotle accepted the morality of exposing infants and supposed that "value" and worth were not intrinsic but acquired.[37] The third century writer Heliodorus felt, contrary to these ancient classical values, that it was not permissible to disregard an "imperiled soul" once it has taken on human form.[38] In the early centuries of the Roman Empire, inspired by Constantine, there developed a growing humanitarianism, a medical ethic of respect for human life, that condemned abortion and active euthanasia. Christians held that "the immortal soul rested in the unborn fetus as truly as in the newborn,"[39] and revered and mourned the death of a fetus. Thus, there flourished a sentiment of altruism and philanthropy with regard to the value of a person, and therefore a capacity for compassion.

Subsequent to primitive and ancient times, there has been reverence for the fetus and newborn, accompanied by the appropriate processes of bereavement, yet there also been irreverence; contrasts of beliefs and rituals abound. At one extreme is infanticide; at the other, a desire for large families and the blessings of fertility.[40] The Dark Ages, later medieval times, and even the Renaissance were among the darkest periods for women and childbearing. Obstetrical practices included cruel and hideous atrocities. So many fetuses and newborns died from disease and obstetrical disasters that to mourn them was felt too burdensome and overwhelming for the families. Evidence of high rates of mortality among children can be seen by observing those buried in medieval English cemeteries. In two such cemeteries, more than 50% of those buried are children, and the largest single category is children aged up to five years.[41] There is also evidence of the burial of fetuses.[42] In contrast to these formalized burials, there existed religious and cultural customs in which funerary rites were not observed for the miscarried fetus, stillborn, or newborn infant. There were "secret (Christian) burials of un-baptized infants . . . excluded from the confines of the church cemetery."[43] Early Jewish law, in an effort to spare parents the "pain" of mourning, restricted acknowledgment of the demise of a fetus or newborn to thirty-one days or more, and these children were not "accorded full human status."[44] The Yoruba tribe in Nigeria would throw a dead baby or stillborn into the bushes, fearing that if the dead baby were buried in the ground, it would offend the shrines of fertility.[45] In contrast, Hindu newborns and stillborns *were* buried, so they might return to an "earthly life."[46]

CHERISHED PURPOSES: SELECTIONS FROM A DOCTOR'S POEMS

Just as despair can be given to me only by another human being,
Hope too can be given to me only by another human being.[1]

Perinatal loss entails a unique bereavement and is an exceptional type of loss. While the death of a baby is a catastrophe and a tragedy that shatters the good, secure, and confident life in a matter of moments, the sharing of feelings of such profound loss with others undergoing similar losses, a community of loss, can beget a healing experience. Healing must take from the despair of our grief its thoughts, memories, and tears, and within a framework of inspiration, introspection, and time, transform this grief into promise and hope. I approach the healing of this penetrating perinatal and neonatal loss experienced by my patients through the use of three modalities:

Healing the spirit through language that is poetry

Healing the loneliness through communication

Healing the body and mind through medical care and information.

What follows are thoughts gleaned from the roots of my soul and written on occasions of death, futility, and desperation; words and poems with dark themes, written with embers of hope amid fires of love—love for my profession and for what I really care about; an attempt to strive for the "happiness of others,"[2] even in their darkest hours. "To know the worst and write in spite of that, that must be love."[3] Poetry and words written from such love, in a muddle of frustration and despair, gather up hope in the art form of language, just as the physician, with stethoscope, scalpel, and pharmacopoeia does in the art form of medicine. Healing thus springs from the

10

complementary remedies of poetry and medicine. Exposing the soul to clear view, the poet speaks by acknowledging weakness. He writes what he feels when he can do no more.

Poems become "words against death."[4] "The poet exploits the cadence of our language"[5] to feed the soul with beauty. The words of the poem not only must "sound" but also must "speak."[6] Y'haudi Amachi, the great Israeli poet, feels "that every poem should be the last poem, written as if it contained the last thing the poet would ever say, shaped to contain the condensation of all the messages of his or her life. It should be a virtual will."[7]

As a physician-poet I write my words—for myself and for my patients—when I have been left without other means of expression. I have lived by the words "cherished purposes" from the time I was a college student in Philadelphia, searching for meaning, for a purpose in my life. Chiseled in a statue memorializing the bravery and the spirit of the soldiers of the Civil War, the words below also came to be chiseled in my mind:

> Each for himself gathered up
> the cherished purposes of life;
> its aims and ambitions;
> its dearest affections;
> and flung all with life itself
> into the scale of battle.
>   Anonymous

I choose to interpret these beautiful words freely and have applied them to my life as standard-bearer for my resolve and commitment to search for meaning. They have been a watchtower for me and are meant as a watchtower for those who must grieve these tragic losses.

Divus

I loved
the quiet time I spent
when every heart beat
you had sent
to my flesh
and to my skin
flowed forth to bring
me peace within
your silent womb,
. . . I loved the silent time.

And even as
my tiny heart
labored at death's call

11

before my start
at birth and life,
and as I ailed,
soon no longer
to inhale
or feel your pulse to mine,
. . . I loved the quiet time.

My body now
apart from yours,
still lives, yet not
upon your shores,
and suffers not
nor is in pain
for within
its new domain
I can love the quiet time.
. . . I loved the quiet time.

Divus is the Latin expression for a Godlike, blessed memory. This poem was written for and given to a patient whom I had not met until she came into labor and was found to have fetal demise.

Erinnyes

What I am, I am.
My afflictions are my affections.
My chaos, civility.
Tides pause, breaths sigh.
Those who dream, dream.
While I with pleasure cast
Ravages and travail obscene,
To a venomous sea, to shatter
Upon the cliffs of despair,
Forgotten forever
As I travel untraveled avenues
Of promise.

In Greek mythology, Erinnyes (or Eumenides) avenged wrongs.

Memnon

My tears are watermarks
Which imprint forever,
Sentient reminders of gentle hopes

And dreams subdued.
Extant in painful thought they are,
And sleep afar
In caves of ancient echoes,
Wailing for my perished child
Who now, guised in angle's silk,
Sings madrigals of sweet delight
And turns my tears heavenward,
To drift peacefully into the
Forgiving canyons of winter's night.

Memnon was the son of Eos, goddess of dawn, who mourned his death by weeping every morning.

Zachary

Where golden swans and princes dance,
My prince has danced and dances still
As my heart with fire burns the pain
And turns its acrid char
To sweet and boundless faith
Which love cements from flesh to flesh to soul,
Dear prince who danced and dances still.

For a newborn who died of multiple congenital anomalies.

Love Contained

Music floats on streams
Of summer's final breath
As rains of hope
Wash famine from my lips.
And now love contained
Within my marrow sleeps,
And I am left to dream and wonder
While angst becomes my silent partner,
Dueling with the rain.
I love the music
Which floats on streams
Of summer's final breath,
And hear it even as
Sadness mutes its song.
For its rhythm is certain
As the pulse of my heart;

Its voice everlasting,
As my memory is long.

This poem was written for twin boys, Andrew and Joseph, who died before birth. It was recited by their courageous parents at their sons' memorial service.

... My Heart Be Yours Forever

I make you both a promise in these my infant days,
Half my heart be yours forever,
The other for God—in praise.
For he has blessed me with abundance,
Granted more than I can give,
Never will I feel dismay. . . . Your love is why I live.
When you hold me very close,
Your pulse feels slow and sure,
Which calms the flutters of my heart
And gives me hope that's pure.
As my parents you are frightened
That my tiny heart is frail,
That my body cannot endure assaults
Fate to it assails.
So I must tell you, mother, father,
I implore you . . . be assured,
Spirit transcends my adversities,
Horizons harbor my cure.

For Sydney, born with a serious congenital heart defect, who survived and is thriving today.

Aoide

The first song on earth
Was a child's cry,
A canticle of absolute beauty.
Each note a bequest for eternity. Ageless
music of heart-sounds
And first-breath sighs
To immortalize
The promise of humankind.

Aoide is the Boeotian muse of song. These lines are dedicated to the labor and delivery suite of Yale-New Haven Hospital, where I practice.

Birth

I have seen the caul,
like honey glazed,
contain and bathe
in sweet succor,
kept watch as
mother's wombs
tear in pain to
bear their child
and then,
as if my first,
stood aside and
cried with awe at
the birth,
that quiescent harbor
where life sings
psalmic verses
of calms and storms,
rains and draughts,
sunlights and dark nights,
agendas to live on forever.

This states as best I can the overwhelming emotion I feel, day after day, as I attend births.

Sonnet of Faith

Appareled in a veil of grace,
Angst and despair showed its face.
Yet from your eyes a gleam did shine,
A hint of nature's grand design
To teach us all that we must cope,
And never lose our faith and hope.
That all things bad and all things sad
Will be eclipsed by what makes us glad:
Love and trust in one another,
Wholesome values as father, mother,
Embracing our children sweet and fair,
Holding their hands, combing their hair.
These are the flames that within us burn,
The passions strong for which we yearn.
So while today your loss brings drear,
The morrow's sunshine will again appear.

Written for a young couple who terminated a pregnancy for a lethal genetic anomaly. They had a wonderful understanding of each other and a devotion to their three-year-old daughter that allowed them to face their bereavement with strength and hope.

Ventose

The chilling winds of March do blow,
As on this day we mourn.
And from our eyes fresh tears do flow,
. . . our child will not be born.
With God's consent did she ascend
To his Empyrean throne,
A refuge surely to transcend
This grief we feel at home.
So as the Ventose winds abate
And springtime flowers bloom,
We know her soul is incarnate
In Heaven's immortal womb.

Empyrean is the highest abode of God. *Ventose*, in French, represents the March winds. This couple's pregnancy terminated in the fourth month, after an infection developed in the uterus.

Pax

Far above the obscure shore
The sky cast forth a darkness visible
That speaks your sadness forever more,
Of a loss that's ever so insensible.
But above these clouds where the sunbeams glow
With no shadows to cast or eclipse,
My soul lives on; I feel no sorrow,
For in my world, I still exist.
To those who love me, I feel your love.
There is no pain, I am at rest.
I have my peace in this heaven above,
And with your prayers I am forever blessed.

Written for parents upon the loss of their son, David.

Cameron

I no longer see the stars; I am the stars.
I no longer breathe the wind; I am the wind.

I am the sweet smell of honeysuckle after an
Evening rain.
I am the dew on the rose petals in early
Morning.

I am harmony and I am peace.
I am love.

In sorrow, my mother and father cry,
But they need not fear. For I am strong.
My heart is whole and in union with my soul.
I understand my fate and I smile.
For nature's will is my destiny
And my guide through eternity.

After his parents' years of infertility, Cameron was born, only to die soon after birth of congenital heart disease. Unlike most forms of congenital heart disease, Cameron's was inoperable and fatal. His courageous parents were with him every moment of his short but love-filled life.

The Rain

Around me falls the silent rain,
Dark clouds sound the thunder.
My body's failed me once again.
Can I endure much more? I wonder.

A weakened mind cries out for mercy,
A stronger heart . . . it quests for hope.
There is no sun—today is dreary,
A shroud of mourning does envelop.

The wrath I sense cannot be stated
In words that one can understand.
All good feelings have now abated,
My tears I wipe with weakened hand.

Fields of lilies grow this spring,
They bloom in all their glory . . .
Yet for me there is no life to bring.
My child is but a memory.

Only despair was felt by this patient, who after two miscarriages and one ectopic (tubal) pregnancy, carried this pregnancy into the 22nd week. Without warning, at a routine visit to my office, it was found that her fetus was dead.

Obstare

I have stood here before
When birth deceived and
Surrendered to my hands
The very spirit and soul of humanity;
The essence of life, save life itself.
And I have touched before
The angel hair and silken skin;
A child lay bare, still and silent
In these outstretched hands
As my will cried out
To scream a breath of life
Into his pale lips
Now frozen in the mist
Of endless dreams.
Yet today I smile
As I have smiled before,
For from such drear
Comes a voice;
A voice, so serene
That it transforms
The searing pain felt in
Our hearts into song;
Melting stones of sorrow
Into liquors of love,
Forever a memory
Of our dear Child.

Obstare is the Latin root for *Obstetrics*, which means "to stand before."

Secret Wonders

Born silent, born still,
With the beauty of an angel,
Elizabeth passed from my waiting hands,
Into the hearts of her parents.
First breath, last breath,
Breathed within

A body full of love;
Youthful, hopeful, anticipating.
Now a body full of sorrow.
Elizabeth . . . a mother's child,
Embraced by three mothers,
Gave tiny footprints, inked mementos of
What might have been.
Yet as with life itself we are
Guided by fleeting moments of
Sweetness remembered
And promises dreamed.
The veil of death's darkness
Will disappear like melting snows
In springtime.
Mercifully, prayers will turn
Cries into song,
Loneliness will fade.
Life will move on.
Elizabeth has touched us all.
But her death will not harm us,
For she has summoned the secret wonders
Of what means *love*.
And we have now become *her* children.

This poem was written for Elizabeth, who was born still on October 28, 1999. The cause was a constriction of her umbilical cord. This is a poem I wrote for Elizabeth, and her parents read it at her funeral service.

Tiferet

In prayer I plead return,
And in dream, awaken!

I fall to stare at gleaned grasses
scattered about forgotten fields,
singed by a senseless lot,
and thirst to cry forever.

Yet,
I will not be draped
in the blanket of loneliness called solitude.
For deaf of song and absent of vision
of who I am and who are my children,
its veil will descend, then disappear.

We are "alive together."

The margin between breath and breathless
is narrow, like twilight and darkness.
Moments of simple thoughts
become ageless memories.
There is triumph to taste,
love to embrace;
havens of hope to inhabit.

Soon, the curtains of chaos
will rise with the setting stars
as memories of joy
bond with joy itself
and I will smile once more,
at last to breathe a painless sigh
of what is love.

Tiferet, in the discourse of Jewish mysticism, is one of the ten Sefirot and
represents beauty, harmony, and truth.

Rivulets

These are days of tears;
Mist from souls of friendship,
Prayers from bottomless hearts.

Love ripples the silence of fear
Like stones dropped in tide-less ponds,
To carry hope beyond infinity
And dance among the sunshine and blossoms
Of ordinary days, while
Waves of virile uncertainties
Spawn rivulets of faith.

Reason probes for reason.

Yet there is elegance
In the threads of our destiny:
Simplicities of truth entwined
With the complexities of why?
Woven from the sweetness of our moments,
They become the fabric of our being.

Transition begets renewal.

As seasons fuse,
Darkness of long winter nights
Becomes an apparition.
Life burgeons, promises mature,
Inspirations thrive and

Fortune ascends on the
Vapors of despair until
despair exists no longer.

Vernalis
Belonging to the Spring

Undaunted, I greet the paradox of spring.
I dream . . . of golden notes
Floating in the silent night.
Joys of breaths and heartbeats
Simple passions of delight
Sing on winds diaphanous,
Of the glory of the bloom
Which never disappointing,
Soon, bathes all beloved
With perfect hope.

It is the season of opulence
When sweetness obscures
Dark halls of winter's lair
And dew upon the grasses
Cast light of morning's hour
Into the windows of the soul
Where fragments of loveliness . . .
Of love, coalesce
Into being,
Magnificence.

PART II
STORIES AND VIEWS

PARENTS' STORIES OF LOSS

Sorrow which is never spoken
Is the heaviest load to bear.[1]

When I read all the stories about all the pain and heartache that is felt worldwide, it saddens me, but in a way comforts me, knowing I am not alone. Strangers we may be, but yet we are connected by a common thread, the loss of a child, and that makes us all soul mates.[2]

The above poignant expression of the value of sharing loss comes from a visitor to my Internet program, *Hygeia*®. Before electronic mail became available, before bereavement support groups became international foundations,[3] the only means for sharing feelings was personal contact with friends and family members, medical personnel, clergy, and bereavement counselors, either alone or in a group setting. Electronic communications, in the form of E-mail, has established itself as an important medium, if not the paradigm, for contemporary communications, in that it enables its users to communicate and share, worldwide, irrespective of geographic borders and demographic differences.

Communications is the web of human society. The structure of a communication system with its more or less well defined channels is in a sense the skeleton of the social body which envelops it. The content of communications is of course the very substance of human intercourse. The flow of communications determines the direction and the pace of dynamic social development.[4]

Although some might argue that communication and conferencing online might disrupt the "socialization and non-verbal cues which accompany face to face conversation—i.e. body language, facial oral expression,"[5] I feel that

Hygeia® and similar online support sites have demonstrated not only the value of electronic communication but also a newly acquired and growing interest in the search for such communication.

We who have lost children are all connected in that way. . . . I never received any counseling, I never read books, I grieve mostly alone and in private, and only in the last month or so have I begun to search the Internet for information/support to help me deal with my loss.[6]

Below are poems and stories and feelings; poignant and personal reflections from parents with whom I have had contact. Some are my patients, some are my friends, and others are visitors to *Hygeia*®. I have chosen not to indentify the sources or my relationship to the parents in order to emphasize the universality of the bereavement process and to protect their privacy. The selections I have chosen reflect most passionately the sense of sorrow that accompanies the devastation of *parenthood lost*, as well as the hope that thankfully follows. I have edited the "stories" so as to concentrate on the *feelings* behind the losses rather than to present a narrative of the pregnancy history and details. For the most part I have omitted the actual diagnosis of the loss (although it might appear evident) but have included all diagnoses, medical definitions, explanations, and insights into the etiologies in the appendixes and glossary. Many other works about pregnancy loss, mostly written by parents who have experienced these losses and caregivers (bereavment counselors, nurses, social workers, and some physicians), have used stories of loss to "tell a story." I have chosen to explore the "feeling" of the stories so the reader may grasp the universality of emotions inherent in these untimely deaths, no matter the cause or medical history. Although I did not set a finite number of stories to include, my intent is to encompass most kinds of perinatal and neonatal loss. Readers who have lost a pregnancy or a child will most likely find a story and/or a feeling very similar, if not identical, to their own. As the stories are read and reread, they appear to become as one, expressing common thoughts and common feelings; sharing common words, phrases, and sentiments that trumpet the pain of each author-parent. Herein rests their value.

The candor with which parents have told their stories and that I bring to this book is painful, yet cathartic. I am grateful to every parent with whom I have had contact and who has contributed to the *true* foundation of this book. Although not identified in this book by name, each parent and each child carries his/her identity in my thoughts. The following poem is dedicated to *all* children who have died in utero, at birth, or soon therafter (and to their parents).

Martyr for Desire

You are my quiet darling.
Your eyes, like morning, burn
The minutes of futility
To contrite hours, turn
Eastward where begins the dance
Of ocean tides, and slumbers still
The famine of our grief, to hide
So deep within my wounded will.
A promise, poisoned from the start,
So brief, without reply or song,
Did graze your spirit in my field.
"Return to me," I cry, I long.
As chaos prods my anguish, yet
Neglecting fortunes in my soul,
Tinted hues of destiny
Are tender thoughts which sorrow stole
From me when first I heard your voice;
Each murmur on your breath that sang
Like harps converging as a choir,
And chimes afar, with passion, rang.
You are my quiet darling
Within a cold and flawless fire,
And I, a prism in the shadows;
A silent martyr for desire.

Jack and Kyle

We became pregnant in October 1996 and were very excited. In November we were told that we would be having twins, which was even more exciting. I was one of six children, and we had talked about having a large family. However, we also wanted to be young parents to all our children, so we were happy to get off to a fast start with twins. By late December, Carmen started having some difficulties with her pregnancy. Her doctor instructed her to rest and reduce her activities, due to a blood clot in her uterus. Though we were concerned, the condition did not seem too serious, and we hoped rest would cause the clot to dissipate.

Subsequent ultrasounds showed the clot getting smaller, so Carmen's doctor allowed her to move around a little more; dinner and a movie would be all right once in a while. In early March, Carmen called her doctor because she noticed some discharge. An ultrasound showed a little funneling of her cervix, but since there was no apparent contracting, she was told to maintain strict bed rest and have a follow-up ultrasound in four days. The follow-up ultrasound showed increased dilation of her cervix. Carmen was admitted to the hospital immediately. The date was March 10, 1997, and she was 22 weeks' pregnant.

At the hospital, we were told Carmen was fully dilated and that birth could occur at any time. We also were told that at 22 weeks of pregnancy, the babies were not viable. However, an ultrasound showed good growth for one of the fetuses, and if they had any chance for survival, Carmen would have to be transported to a level III hospital. Despite being pregnant with twins and enduring some minor difficulties along the way, it never occurred to us that our babies could be born this early, let alone with little chance for survival. Jack Michael was born on March 13, 1997, and the three days leading up to his birth were the longest three days of our lives.

At the tertiary care hospital, we were awake almost twenty-four hours a day. The daily routine involved meeting with doctors to discuss what would happen if the babies were born this day. As each day passed, their chances for survival would increase; their best chance for survival would be after 24 weeks' gestation. With two weeks until then, it seemed like a lifetime to us. I was distraught, thinking that Carmen would have to lie flat on her back with her feet elevated and be subjected to all these different medications for two weeks, or longer. At the beginning of each shift, the new team of doctors met with us. They provided us with all sorts of statistics regarding probability for survival. Based on this information, which was totally foreign to us, we had to decide what we wanted the doctors to do if our babies were delivered. I remember saying to myself that I could never imagine that at age thirty we would have to be making these kinds of life-and-death decisions about our own children. It was like an entire lifetime was condensed into these three days.

Since this was our first pregnancy, we did not know what to expect. At first we felt anxious but optimistic. We figured that since Carmen was in the hospital under twenty-four-hour care, delivery could be delayed. Initially, we even had thoughts that she might make it to term. As reality set in, we realized there was only so much that doctors could do. Most measures for delaying delivery at this stage are designed to buy you days, maybe weeks, not months. We were now just hoping that they would make it past 24 weeks, or as close to 24 weeks as possible, since all the statistics showed the likelihood of survival jumped exponentially after 24 weeks. It became apparent to us that there was a sort of crossover point, maybe toward the end of 23 weeks' gestation, after which the doctors would recommend increased intervention once the babies are delivered. Before that, however, they were primarily recommending comfort and convalescence. This was very hard for us to understand. As lay people, we could not see how a few more days in the womb could make such a difference in our babies' chances. To us, it was like, if you recommend increased intervention tomorrow, why not today? I remember feeling so angry and frustrated over not knowing what was the best thing to do. The doctors were talking about all these statistics and probabilities, and all I could think was, this is our child we are talking about.

During the three days leading up to Jack's delivery, which seemed like weeks, friends and relatives were giving us information and advice on what to do. Not only had we never contemplated the possibility of premature delivery, we had never realized that many friends, or friends of friends, had similar experiences to share. While the support was a blessing, all the different stories we were hearing about this baby or that baby that had been born at 22 or 23 weeks and was supposedly doing fine only complicated our daily decision on what intervention to request from the doctors. I remember just praying that our babies would make it past 24 weeks' gestation, so that we would not have to make the decision of what to do if they were born sooner.

Our first son was born on March 13, 1997, at 22 weeks and 6 days' gestation. We were praying for the best but expecting the worst. What became important to us as we entered the delivery room was that we be able to baptize him immediately in case he did not survive. Baptism materials were set up in the delivery room. However, when he was delivered, the team of neonatologists whisked him away for examination and assessment. The initial assessment offered hope, but only time would tell how he reacted to the oxygen treatment.

Amazingly, Carmen stopped contracting after he was delivered. Earlier that day, we discussed the possibility of this happening with our doctor. We waited in the delivery room for a very anxious fifteen minutes or so to confirm that the contractions had stopped. Once things calmed down, we wheeled Carmen back to her room. It was like we were in a dream. We could not believe how surreal this all was. We had just gone through delivery of a child, and now Carmen was back in her room resting—and still pregnant.

We had names picked out for both girls and boys. We did not know the sexes ahead of time. The first choice for a boy was Jack Michael. We both loved the name Jack, and Carmen could not wait to call our son by that name. We did not tell the hospital our name choice right away; he was known as Baby A. We considered giving him a different name than Jack. Given the circumstances of his delivery, we considered naming him after Carmen's younger brother, who had died a few years earlier. After thinking about it some more, we decided that since Jack was the name we had chosen for our first son, we should stick with that name. We felt that if we gave him a different name, it would be like admitting we did not think he would survive. We could not bear to give up hope yet.

Our families had been in the waiting room. When I went to tell them of Jack's delivery and to explain how we had to wait and see how he responded to the oxygen, a feeling of love and pride rushed through me as I was talking about my son. I was a father. We were new parents, and despite all the trauma in getting to that point and all the uncertainty ahead of us, we felt happiness in having a son. We thought that as each hour passed, his chances for survival would increase. No news was good news. Then, several hours later, Jack's doctors told us that he was not responding to his medications and that X-rays showed his lungs were not developed enough. Our son would not survive. He was basically living on the respirator.

We had decided earlier not to exert any extraordinary measures to keep him alive; he had been through enough. As much as we wanted him to survive, we did not want him to suffer any more with all the machines and wires hooked up to him. The hardest thing for me that day was to tell our families the news. After describing to them how Jack's condition worsened throughout the day, the hardest part was telling them that Carmen and I decided to have the doctors turn off the machines. I could barely get the words out. After all we had been through over the past three days, it was only now that we fully realized that we would not be bringing our son home. I could not remember a sadder moment in my life.

The doctors and nurses, who were incredibly caring and gracious, wrapped Jack in a blanket and brought him to us to hold before he died. Jack was only 12 1/2 inches long and weighed 1 pound, 5 1/2 ounces, but he was the most beautiful little boy with perfect features, just as if he were full term. It was incredible. We were so happy, for lack of a better word, to be able to hold him and to tell him we loved him, and to say good-bye before he died.

Carmen and I held each other and cried. We could not believe that we were grieving the loss of our son.

The grieving could not last long, at least for now. Carmen was still pregnant, and we had to focus all our energy on her and our second son. It was a miracle to us that the second baby did not deliver with Jack, and it gave us hope that maybe we could make it past 24 weeks. We were told that delayed birth does not happen often, and delivery could occur at any time. But as each hour passed, our spirits were lifted. As we got closer to 24 weeks' gestation, we prayed for one more day, one more day, since we now understood what a difference each day could make to the survival chances of our baby. In addition to the emotional strain on us both, the physical strain on Carmen was enormous. She was subjected to all kinds of medicines designed to delay labor and had to lie in bed all day with the foot of the bed tilted up. To find some humor in this, we talked about how despite all the medical technology, we were relying primarily on gravity to keep our baby inside his mother for as long as possible.

After enduring the side effects of all the medicine for a few days, Carmen was worn out. We decided that it could not possibly be good for our baby if his mother was feeling so lousy. So Carmen stopped taking any medicine designed to stop labor, except for small doses of nifedipine, and we were resolved to accept the fact that whatever happened was meant to happen. Almost immediately, Carmen felt much better. She continued her bed rest, and we again began a game of wait and see. Since the baby was now past 24 weeks' gestation, and therefore was considered viable by our doctors, we were relieved that at least we did not have to decide whether or not to intervene and support the baby's life after delivery. However, an ultrasound indicated the baby was breech. Now we had to decide whether to risk a natural delivery or to do a cesarean section, as the doctors recommended. Given the gestational age, the cesarean would have to be a classical cut, which is more intrusive and harder on the mother, and would have to be repeated for all future deliveries. With Jack's death weighing on our minds, our optimism over the outcome of his sibling's delivery, if it came anytime soon, was weakened. Without really knowing what to do, we decided that this was in God's hands, and if this baby was meant to survive, it would. And if it wasn't then we could accept that, but we did not want to subject Carmen's body to a classical cut cesarean in the process. The next thing that happened can only be described as a miracle, and I still tell the story with amazement.

Carmen went into labor on March 26, 1997, in the early evening, thirteen days after Jack had been delivered. It started out being pretty routine: push-relax, push-relax. The primary concern was that once Carmen's water broke, the birth canal might collapse onto the baby, causing its head to get stuck as it passed through the canal, and cutting off its oxygen. The miracle was that the water did not break until the baby was literally halfway outside Carmen's body. When it finally did break, the baby just shot out into the doctor's arms from the force of the water breaking. Our second son, Kyle Mark, was born at nearly 25 weeks' gestation.

The preliminary prognosis for Kyle was positive, so we were cautiously optimistic. Kyle was in the Newborn Intensive Care Unit (NICU) for fifteen weeks. He was released on July 11, 1997, his scheduled due date. Kyle's stay in the NICU was a roller-coaster ride for him and for us. After Carmen's release from the hospital, which was delayed a week due to an infection in her uterus, she spent almost every day at Kyle's side. We lived one hour from the hospital, and I would visited most nights and on weekends. At first, while Kyle was in an incubator, we could hardly touch him for risk of infection. We prayed, sang songs, and read books to Kyle so he could hear our voices. It was the most helpless feeling, knowing that our child was struggling for life and feeling we could do so little to help him. We did not really feel like parents, because even though we visited Kyle whenever we could, at the end of the visit we returned home without him. Even though Kyle survived his delivery, he was still so small and premature that he was not out of the woods yet. All the while, our son Jack was still in the morgue at the hospital. We wanted to have a burial service for Jack, but knowing that we could not go through that twice, we could not do it until we were sure that Kyle was going to make it. As time passed, and the chances of Kyle's survival increased, we were still concerned about how he would grow developmentally.

All we wanted was a happy and healthy baby, and while he seemed fine in the hospital, there was really no way for us to know for sure what problems might become apparent as he got older. There are so many ups and downs, in the NICU, regarding not only your own child but also other families and their children. You are there so often, you can't help bonding with others experiencing the same heartache. The worst experience was witnessing the loss of a child by other parents and, while grieving for them, being reminded that your child is not out of the woods yet. We have formed friendships with other parents that I am sure will last forever. Strong bonds are made when you share such a difficult part of your lives together. I know those bonds helped us endure some long nights at the hospital.

As Kyle's condition improved steadily, we were allowed to hold him more and eventually became more involved with his daily care, including bathing, feeding, and holding him while he slept. We became so excited by each little milestone, whether it was drinking a full bottle—which for him was less than an ounce—or the day he was moved from the incubator to an open bassinet. We could finally touch him without reaching through holes. The struggle was so long and hard that even little accomplishments were major events for us.

Another emotional struggle was our wanting to remember our son Jack.

All our energy was focused on Kyle while he was in the hospital, so we did not have a chance to stop and remember Jack. Our friends and family did not always know what to say or do. It was a strange circumstance: saddened over the loss of a son while happy over the birth of another, but still concerned that he too might not survive or, if he did, with what ailments. We finally had a burial service for Jack in May 1997. We never thought that at age thirty, we would be picking out a burial site for our son.

Finally, on July 11, 1997, his expected due date, Kyle was discharged from the hospital. We were so excited to be finally taking him home, but at the same time incredibly nervous about not having the support of the nurses and heart monitors. We had become so reliant on the monitors that I was seriously concerned that I would not be able to tell if he was breathing while he slept. He weighed about 4 1/2 pounds when he came home. He was so fragile, we were afraid to let anyone touch him. Also, his lungs were still premature, and we had to be careful about exposure to others, to avoid even minor colds.

Kyle is almost two years old now, and doing beautifully. But the hardest thing to deal with since he came home, and even today, is having to treat him differently because he was so premature. For the first year we could barely take him out in public for fear of his getting sick. As parents, it is frustrating to see other kids who are the same age as Kyle and are bigger and more developed. While we are truly blessed by his progress, we want so much for our child to fit in unnoticed with his age group, so he doesn't grow up thinking he is different in any negative way.

We talk to Kyle about his brother Jack and someday hope to share the whole story with him. We worry that he might feel guilty that his brother died and he lived. Seeing Kyle grow and develop has been a wonderful experience. Now that we are approaching his second birthday, we look at Kyle and wonder what life would have been like had Jack survived. Would they look alike? Would they have similar personalities? Would they play well together and grow up being best friends? Though Kyle gives us so much joy, it saddens us to know that they won't know each other. We bring Kyle to the cemetery, which is just down the street from our house, to visit Jack. And when we drive by, which is often, we wave and blow kisses to Jack and say, "Hi, Jack, we love you!"

We want to keep Jack's memory alive for our sake and for Kyle's. It is sometimes difficult to do. Our families and friends pay so much attention to Kyle and give him so much love, that they sometimes don't remember or acknowledge that he had a brother. We have to remember that just because he did not live a very long life, that doesn't mean he is any less loved or missed.

We certainly hope never to go through an experience like this again. But remembering that it was Kyle who has had to endure the most through all this causes our love for him to be that much stronger. We have been blessed with a beautiful son here on earth and a beautiful son watching over us from heaven. While we would give anything to have both of them here with us, we still, in many ways, consider ourselves to be the luckiest parents in the world.

As of December 1998, Kyle weighs about twenty-three pounds and is about thirty-one inches tall. He is a very happy little boy. He loves meeting new people, especially other children, and listening (and dancing) to music. He also loves animals, especially dogs. His pediatrician is very pleased with his progress, and so are we.

A Mother's Loss: Found

The pain, the pain that can't be seen, the pain that never leaves me, the cut that never heals. This is what I feel when I think back to that time, the time my son was born. There is a lot of pain associated with this birth and death; feelings never dealt with; feelings never validated, worthlessness.

It was not bad enough that I was not worth anything to anyone else or to myself in the earliest years of my life—or so I was made to feel; this loss of my son and the way I was treated further instilled the belief that I was worthless for many years. So many years, until I was much older and wiser and worked at my worth within myself, without the validation of others.

They just took him from me. I know I heard a cry. They said it was my imagination. I begged that he be baptized. I still don't know if they did that. I begged them to keep him warm. I still don't know if they even heard me. I told them to tell him I loved him. I don't know if he was told. They covered my eyes. I wanted to see, but the drugs took the fight out of me. I gave in to the bliss of the painless, drug-induced blackness and wanted it to all go away. But it didn't go away. It still hasn't. I awoke to the face of a doctor I did not know standing over me. He said, ". . . can you hear me?" How strange, I thought, calling me by my first name and he didn't know me. He came only to tell me, "Your son expired shortly after 6 P.M. Would you or your husband like to go down and see him?" How personal, I thought, him calling me by name—and how cold to tell me my son "expired." I was so confused at this warm personalization mixed with detachment. How it got me, in the pit of my empty spot where he used to be. I didn't go. My husband went and came back and told me how beautiful he was, that he looked like me. I wanted to hold my son. I was never told I could. I was crying after everyone left that night, only to be told by the nurse, "Don't be so hard on yourself, honey, it could be worse. The woman down the hall lost twins last night." Then I was given a sedative, and that was it. I guess losing two babies made it worse somehow, and I should be ashamed that I had lost only one child!

I hurt all over, even inside, where no one could see. The core of me, the one that held secrets, the secret that my husband beat me just two days before I lost my son and I didn't dare blame him. No, I couldn't—I would get hit again—so I stuffed the hurt of the loss and my resentment toward my husband.

The social worker gave me some papers to sign the next morning. I said, "I want to wait for someone to read these with me." She said, "Oh, that's not necessary; they just say that you don't want an autopsy on the baby." I said "OK," and signed. To this very day I don't know what I signed. I just believed and trusted her. I went home the next day with breasts on fire and my body sore, physical reminders that I had given birth but had nothing to show for it except an empty place in my heart and soul never to be filled again. They said they would bury him for us, but I could never know where. I didn't question. I was scared to question. I don't know why. I had a four-year-old at home who needed me. I made the mistake of thinking they would put some worth on my son's body and would treat it with dignity. Again I trusted.

It has been twenty-four years now, and I've grown strong as a person and a woman. I have found out where my son is buried. With the love and support of a lot of wonderful, generous people I have had a memorial stone put in his place of burial and of all the babies who never had a chance at life—maybe even those twins the nurse told me about. This memorial can serve for all children, not just there but the abused, forgotten children all over the world who need to be validated as worthwhile human beings. I have come full circle and I feel joy, not sorrow, at the sight of this beautiful place where he rests. It is a place to come and celebrate his coming into the world and leaving it so quickly. It reminds me daily that I will see him again when my time comes, and I can tell him then, face to face, what I know he feels from my heart today: that I loved him then and I love him now.

The grief I felt at the moment . . . was beyond words. . . . I sobbed until my heart could cry no more. For years I carried this sadness deep inside.

Sarah

My name is Jennifer. My daughter, Sarah, was stillborn. If anyone had told me two years ago that I would be writing these words, I would not have believed them. The death of a child is such an unbelievable event that I know you, too, are in shock that it has happened to you. I have written a book, *Letters to Sarah*, with the hope of easing some of the pain and of informing others of what lies ahead.

In my ninth month of pregnancy, my friends from college threw a baby shower for me. About two hours before the shower, Sarah kicked over a hundred times. This was unusual. I had never done fetal movement counts, but this one time, I stopped to count because I knew the baby was kicking more than ever before. Daniel felt the kicks as well. Throughout the shower, we commented to our friends on how strong this baby was. Those were the last kicks I ever felt.

During the first twenty-four hours without movement, I figured, "Well, he/she is just worn out from earlier." But by the second day, I was getting worried. I dug out a stethoscope to listen for a heartbeat. I had always been able to find it before, but this time, I could hear only the echo of my own heart. I said nothing to Daniel. We went shopping and made plans. That night I pulled out the stethoscope once again, with no result. The following morning I told Daniel that I believed the baby had died. He then got out the stethoscope and "found" a heartbeat. I wanted so badly for him to be right that I allowed myself to be comforted for the time being.

The baby appeared to have dropped, so I told myself he/she is too crowded to move. When I mentioned a lack of movement to others, they supplied the same hope. Finally, I went to the doctor. He had difficulty locating a heartbeat, but he did eventually "find" one. He then sent me to the main hospital. The nurses searched for a heartbeat and did not find one. My panic was rising, and when the doctor arrived with a portable ultra-sound, he confirmed my worst fear. The baby had been dead for several days.

I chose to induce labor but asked them to wait until Daniel could arrive. I had to call him from the hospital to utter the horrible words, "The baby died, but I still have to go through labor and delivery." Sitting in the hospital room, waiting to get this over with, was the worst experience of my life. The hospital was at least a four-hour drive for Daniel.

When he finally arrived, we cried together and prepared for the long night ahead. I was given painkillers on request and spent much of the time "out of it." Sarah was delivered after twenty-one hours of labor. I chose to see her before consenting to drugs. I will never regret this decision. I was able to hold her, but Daniel only got to see her, kiss her forehead, and say "I love you, Sarah." He then left the room.

I partially unwrapped the blanket to look at her, but I felt as if I was being watched and that this was inappropriate. I never thought to ask to be alone with her or for Daniel to return before sending her away. She was perfect-looking, lots of black hair, a round face, and long, beautiful fingernails. She weighed 7 pounds, 1 ounce, and looked normal.

The funeral was planned by my parents, and the nursery was dismantled while I was away. Sarah was buried in my hometown with a graveside service. Friends from college attended or sent flowers. I was numb, amazed that any of this was taking place. I just wanted to be strong and get on with my life. I felt that this was what was expected of me.

It was not until the day Daniel, as well as my mother and twin sister, had to return to work that I was alone to think. Then it hit me how much I loved Sarah and how much I had lost. I cried uncontrollably all day. I could not understand. "Why?" "What did I do to deserve this?" "What is wrong with me?" "Why didn't she love me enough to stay?" Two weeks later, I returned to classes and was treated like a glass doll. I felt as if everyone was looking at me and saying "She's the one with the dead baby." I faced people who tried to help but those comments were hurtful. I tried to turn off my pain, appear strong and "get over it," but deep inside, I was hurting more and more each day. I eventually realized that denying my grief was only going to prolong it.

Difficult Decisions

They told us our baby had two cysts on the brain, thickening of the neck, and only three chambers of the heart; an amniocentesis revealed trisomy 18. It was a very hard decision, but we had to be strong and supportive in the decision we made to interrupt the pregnancy when I was 20 weeks along. It was the hardest decision to make because we have waited so long and tried so hard to become pregnant. When our daughter was born, we weren't sure if we wanted to see her, hold her, or anything. I was so scared. When she was born, I knew I had to be strong to see what had been kicking me from the inside. We held her, named her, got photos of her, handprints and footprints. I cherish everything I have. Now that I look back, I would have regretted not doing the things I did. We then had to bury her, so we got her the best headstone we could find. We love her dearly.

Love

Our son died last year. We chose, in a decision filled with horror, anguish, pain, and *love*, to have an abortion after learning that our son had defective kidneys and was in the early stages of congestive heart failure. I was just shy of 20 weeks' pregnant. I still miss him every day. I started out this grieving process feeling mostly sad, missing my baby, and have progressed through many other feelings, including anger, helplessness, fear. I have played around with acceptance, but I don't think I'm there yet! In addition to our sorrow over our lost baby, we learned not long after the abortion that the disease he had is a hereditary one. I really want to be a mother, and to carry our own child, but it is beyond frightening to think of having to have a second or third abortion of a baby that I want; that I love and cherish. I have had an early miscarriage since the abortion, and while this loss caused some sadness and frustration, it was nothing at all like having to make the decision to end the baby's life.

Our Son

Our son was born on February 11, 1993, and died two hours and twenty-seven minutes later. He was beautiful. He was 3 pounds, 2 3/4 ounces, and took a deep breath and cried a loud cry when he was born. I think when he cried, both my husband and I thought he would be OK. He died a peaceful death in my arms. People ask me how I could have him die in my arms and say that it would be too difficult for them to do; my answer was that I was his mother, and he knew I was holding him. He could feel my heart beating, and I certainly wasn't going to let him die in a stranger's arms or on a little cot in a corner of a room by himself. This was going to be the only and last thing I could ever do for my child, and I was determined not to let him down. Two days later we buried our son. I think that out of all of this, this was the hardest thing I had to do both emotionally and physically. You are supposed to bring your child home to a warm, cozy crib, not put him in a casket in the cold ground. For some reason, I have a hard time dealing with this. The night he was buried, I took a hot bath. As I was lying in the tub that night, my breast milk started to come in. It was so ironic. There was no baby to nurse. How could God be so cruel, I thought. Some people abuse their children and don't want to become pregnant—I, on the other hand, wanted another child to be a part of our family, and I couldn't have him. Of course there have been lots of feelings and emotions in the last four years, and I think that it's only now that I have the emotional strength to talk about him. I long to hold him in my arms just one more time, but I have to think that he is our little angel in Heaven. We openly talk about him now and even sign cards with his name. I got a Mother's Day card yesterday and his name was included. I think that keeping your child a part of your family helps with the grief.

My Son

    I would like to share my feelings, hoping that it will give me some peace. I awoke to realize that my baby wasn't moving the way he usually did in the morning. Somehow I just knew my baby was gone. An ultrasound revealed our worst fears. I will never forget seeing that little, still heart on the ultrasound screen. We went home and held each other and cried. The next morning I told our other children, and we began the awful process of trying to induce our baby to leave my womb. Finally I delivered my son with his umbilical cord tightly wrapped twice around his little neck. I held him and cried for all that we had lost and for this precious little life that had been cut short before it ever began. Two days later we buried him under a beautiful tree with chimes blowing in the wind.

My Precious Daughter

My precious daughter was born during the 19th week of my pregnancy. She had spina bifida. We were devastated and heartbroken beyond imagination. She would be paralyzed from the waist down and would most likely have bowel and bladder problems, hydrocephalus, and unknown mental disabilities. Although we were in total shock, we pulled ourselves together and tried to figure out what we should do and tried to learn as much about spina bifida as we could. What was the best thing for our baby? I don't think I'll ever know for sure what the right thing was—there is no "right" answer in a situation like this. No one wins. There is no happy ending. With much sadness, my husband and I decided to end the pregnancy. Although this was the most traumatic thing I have ever gone through, some good came out of it. The nurses and doctors were absolutely wonderful and compassionate, especially, the genetic counselor who helped us through it all. She convinced me that I might want to see my baby. I treasure the few moments I had with my daughter after the delivery and am so thankful for having had the chance to see and hold her. That moment is etched in my memory forever.

The hospital prepared a "birth" certificate, made footprints, and took two photographs. These items, along with my daughter's blanket and cap, are kept in a special keepsake bag. I felt so very sad for our poor little girl. She was so ill. My arms ached for her as they wheeled me out of the hospital. It felt so strange. I was pregnant, and now I'm not. There is no baby to take home and care for, love, and hold. She was buried in the baby section of a beautiful cemetery the following Monday. We had a short memorial service and several family members attended. She was buried with a stuffed animal my sister gave me when she found out I was pregnant, a picture of my husband and me, and a picture of our two dogs. My husband and I visit the grave often. It has now been nine months, and my husband and I have been up and down emotionally. I've told others who have asked that we will never forget our baby; the pain just eases as time goes by; and the good days start to outnumber the bad as you pass through the stages of grief. We have thought about having another baby, but we've lost our "innocence" and realize that another pregnancy right now would be filled with fear and worry about it happening again (our chance of recurrence is about 5%). We haven't given up on the idea completely; we just want to wait a while longer.

My Pretty Little Girl

In memory of my second born daughter, Alison Hannah McMahon. I still feel the pain.

Since your birth twelve years ago
There has never been a day when I haven't thought of you
I have hurt every day for the loss of you
And still I cannot let you go
I want to have you back in my arms
There are so many things I have wanted to share with you
teach you, laugh or cry about with you
Sadly I have lived through these years still grieving
I ache so much to have lost you
I was so happy and proud to have brought you into the world
Then I had to let you go
I thought I would die the pain was so raw and deep
It always seems like yesterday to me
Even now I can feel you in my arms
That small, beautiful girl I longed to bring home to love
My love is always yours, Today, Tomorrow, Forever

Rosebud

I realized I hadn't felt movement. I had two separate dreams that my baby had died, so when I went into the hospital, I wasn't surprised when no heartbeat could be found. I was induced, and gave birth to a beautiful, perfect daughter. There is no indication of why she died (even after the autopsy). We brought her home with us for the weekend, and she was buried on a bed of rose petals with the casket surrounded by white rosebuds, which people who came to the funeral had brought. She is our little rosebud blooming in heaven. Now, five months later, our life has hardly changed (outwardly) from before I became pregnant. Inwardly our life has changed considerably, and for the better. The experience has enabled us to get close to our families and to God. It has strengthened our love for each other and for the world we live in. It has given us more confidence in ourselves; we've survived a very traumatic event intact. We can survive anything. Most people probably find our philosophy strange (I do), but I've found that my faith that this is part of God's great plan, which we can't understand but can trust, has helped me heal. My faith does not heal the pain in my arms at not having a baby to hold, or the pain in my heart when I see my friends' babies, or the pain of being back at work when I want to be at home with a baby. But it does help with the question Why us?

A Lasting Pain

I have not been able to write down my experience until now because it is just too raw and too painful. I have not wanted to dig so deeply into myself and revisit the most painful experience of my life. Even to begin writing it just cuts me to the core, yet there has not been a day since this happened that I do not think about it. There is constant pain. Even as I write this, I feel the tears coming, and my chest hurts and my belly hurts. Prior to this I did not know that grief physically hurts.

I did not grieve after the first miscarriage. I told myself that it is just one of those things, and because the relationship I was in at that time was not sound, that it was not meant to be. I got on with my life and was back at work within a week.

My princess was born breathing and alive. I heard her whimper as the staff rushed her to the corner of the room and began working on her. It was the only time I heard her voice. She weighed 1 pound, 7 ounces. She was beautiful. Tiny but perfectly formed. She had black curly hair peeping out from the hat she had on. She was connected to machines and tubes and monitors, and was on a ventilator. We held her hand and welcomed her to the world.

The next morning we went in to see her, and it hit me just how tiny she was. Her whole arm was the size of my big finger; her chest was the size of my hand. The doctors said that she was doing well; her chances were good. They told us black girls had the greatest survival records. I began expressing breast milk, and she was fed by a tube through her nose; 1 milliliter at first, and then she got up to 5 milliliters every three hours within a few days. By that weekend I began to feel robbed, as if the womb snatchers had struck. I felt empty and hollow.

I had my baby but I did not have her. I could not hold her, feed her, or anything, but I was grateful that she was alive. The level of oxygen she was receiving was reduced. Then she developed an infection. They did not know what it was but started treatment. Her oxygen was increased again. Then there seemed to be some improvement. She was started again on breast milk. They weighed her, and after a week she had gone up to 1 pound, 13 ounces; she looked bigger to us. Her condition began to fluctuate. She would be OK for a few days, then something would happen. I could not leave her, for I was afraid that if I left her, she would feel abandoned and die. So I stayed with her. I would sit with her all day every day, and sing to her and talk to her and wash her and change her diaper and just love her. I told her secrets, I told her of our plans for her, and our dreams. I told her about her family. I fed her through the tube. I washed her body with a cotton ball. I oiled her skin. I kissed her fingers. I believe she knew I was her mommy and I was there. Her daddy came and sang to her and talked to her. She knew him and always opened her eyes when he spoke.

They needed to transfer my daughter to another hospital because she became much sicker. I prayed so hard, Please don't let her die, please don't let me have known her for five weeks, just for her to be taken away now. Just don't let her die. I prayed, If there is really a God, grant me this one thing and I will never again ask for anything. We refused to accept that she was going to die. I whispered in her ears: "Baby, Mommy and Daddy love you. When you have had enough, you stop. I want you here with me, but if it hurts too much, you stop. I will understand."

I could not watch her suffer anymore. The doctors told us there was nothing else they could do for her and that we should consider switching off the ventilator. We spoke with our families and loved ones in the waiting room (there must have been about twelve family members there), and together we made the decision that enough was enough. I was so glad they were there to help us make that decision, because I could not have made it alone. We agreed to switch off the machines.

We had a naming ceremony for her. Everyone held her and kissed her and wept. Then her dad and I took her into the parents' room where we had been staying, and I held her to my chest. For the first and last time I felt her naked skin against my naked skin. We took pictures and hugged together for about fifteen minutes. My precious baby girl died on my chest. My world fell apart and I changed forever. She had a beautiful burial ceremony with about 150 people (family, friends, and loved ones) in attendance. We were fortunate that we were able to bring her body home for two nights. We kept her on ice. Maybe some people will think that is morbid, but to me there is nothing morbid about my baby. She was ours. We wanted her to know where home would have been. I carried her around the house and showed her her room and the things I had prepared for her. I made her a beautiful outfit to be buried in, and my sister and her dad made the casket and lined it with yellow satin. In the casket with her we put gifts from her aunties and uncles and toys and photographs.

Now, eight months later, it hurts as much as it did on the night she died. It does not go away. I am not the same person anymore. I feel like such a failure. It is the most natural thing in the world to have a child, yet I could not carry my baby to term. She was born only to suffer and die.

Who feels it, knows it. Nothing can compare to your child dying. Sometimes I wish I had died with her. It is only now that I can go to the cemetery and not feel like digging up the grave with my bare hands, just so that I can see her again. I know I have changed, and I long to feel normal again.

How can something that is supposed to bring such joy just bring so much pain and sorrow? I feel jealous when I see happy young mothers with babies . . . I feel so angry when I hear moms complaining that their baby kept them awake that night. Oh, for that pleasure I would give everything. . . . People don't want to hear about this all the time, but I still want to talk about her. They don't understand what it feels like to know I never heard her call me Mommy. I never heard her crying or laughing. . . . I'll never comb her hair or comfort her. Yes, I am a mother! But my baby is not here with me.

My Grief

I was 22 weeks' pregnant with a baby boy when a routine ultrasound revealed two major congenital heart defects. All of our previous genetic and ultrasound exams had been completely normal, so I was not expecting any problems of this magnitude. To my shock, the pediatric cardiologist began discussing the possibility of terminating the pregnancy. After long and tearful discussions with my husband and our families and friends, we decided to terminate the pregnancy. I had an abortion in my 23rd week of pregnancy. It has been almost two years since our baby died. I still cry easily and often. In thinking about our baby recently, I realized that a good deal of the ongoing pain comes from the way our baby died. I feel as though I abandoned him at the moment of his death. One moment I was pregnant and the next I wasn't. It was an unbelievable shock. There is a huge disconnection between my experience of time and emotion. I grieve that I was not with him at the time of his death. I could not see him or hold him in my arms. I was unconcious at the time my son, whom I had loved and nurtured for months, died. At the time no one offered me the option of inducing labor and allowing my son to die after birth. I thought about it but did not ask anyone if this was an option; the thought was just too painful. I wish I could have held him as he died. I wish I could have seen him, and spoken to him, and comforted him.

My Twins

After two miscarriages, when I became pregnant again I was worried I'd miscarry again, but I began to relax after the first trimester. Then at 20 weeks we found out I was having identical twin boys. We were very excited and things were going well until 36 weeks, when one baby showed signs of distress. I was monitored closely, and they decided to induce labor the next week. When I showed up at the hospital for the induction, they could find only one heartbeat. It was confirmed by ultrasound that one baby had died (only about two hours earlier). Later that afternoon I delivered twin boys. My first was stillborn, my second was very ill and was transferred to another hospital. They were later diagnosed with a CMV infection. My second boy eventually got better, although we are still dealing with the long-term effects of the infection. I suffered a lot of guilt and depression after my first son's death, almost to the point of being suicidal. But eventually I learned to accept his death and to try to go on with my life. Now it's been almost two years, and I'm expecting another baby soon.

My Son

In the seventh month of my pregnancy I went to the doctor, as I did every month. I had always looked forward to my doctor's appointment to be sure the baby was doing well. I was scheduled for an ultrasound that day, and I was excited to get a glimpse of my baby. While I was on the table, the radiologist began to observe the baby, checking for all his little baby parts and to see if he were growing well. As he proceeded with the test, he began to hesitate. Something was wrong! He had found an absence of amniotic fluid around the baby, and my heart was crushed as he searched again and again for the baby's kidneys. There was none! My husband drove me to the university hospital center. My daughter stayed at her grandma's house, not knowing what was wrong with her baby brother. Upon arrival at the University Medical Center, I felt assured that if anything could possibly be done, it could be done there. I was admitted at once and taken to the maternity ward. The nurses seemed to know we were coming.

They appeared to be nervous around me, and I could feel their tension. I sensed that they knew more than I had been told. After repeated ultrasounds and other tests, we heard the words we hoped we would never hear. Our baby was going to die! He was given a 5% chance of survival. I wanted to collapse. I became totally immobilized. I just knew my heart had shattered, and I was too weak to pick up the pieces. I began to analyze my life for anything I had done wrong that could have caused this to happen. The questions became repetitive. Why me? Why? Our choices were to carry him to full term, giving him his 5% chance of survival, or to induce labor right then. To us there was only one choice; we knew we had to give him a chance. In the month ahead, we were still in a state of shock. My husband and I prayed constantly. We wanted to mourn, but felt it would cause us to lose hope. We were not going to give up and just accept the obvious.

Then on the last day of May, eight months into the pregnancy, I delivered a 4-pound, 11-ounce baby boy. He was taken immediately to intensive care, where they proceeded to resuscitate him. My husband was allowed to visit him shortly after his birth while I was taken to the recovery room to await his diagnosis.

Then the news came. My son was born with Potter's Syndrome, a rare disease that causes the kidneys to not develop. He was not going to survive. I was taken to intensive care on a stretcher to say hello and good-bye to my son. He was beautiful, he looked normal, and I wanted to pick him up and take him home. He looked like his father. He was being kept alive by machines, to allow my husband and me more time with him. He had already begun to suffer, and we were soon asked for permission to disconnect the machines. We were told that once his life support was discontinued, he would die within moments. We were given a private room, and baby's respirator was removed. We held him in our arms and rocked him. We begged and pleaded with God to let him survive. My husband and I were willing to sacrifice our own lives to let this little one live. For two hours my son gasped for breath. He tried to cry but couldn't, because the respirator had damaged his throat. I had never felt more helpless in my life. It felt as though my insides were ripped to shreds as I watched my son take his last breath. The pain is still felt when I think of my beautiful son. All we have left are pictures, a lock of his hair, and the little T-shirt he wore that day. But I learned something through this difficult time. I wasn't angry with God because of my son's death, but thankful for the time he had given us together. Most of all, I was especially proud to be his mother. He was too good for this old world, and he is much better off where he is.

Two years after I buried my son, I gave birth to twins, a boy and a girl. God knew I would never forget my first son, but he found a way to ease my pain. We now have five healthy and beautiful children.

My Daughter

Our daughter, beautiful and precious, was born in August 1998. She was only 21 weeks' gestation. After a level 2 ultrasound and an amnio, she was diagnosed with trisomy 18. We went to genetic counseling and were told that her disorder was incompatible with life. If she were to make it to term, she would have had a life full of pain and suffering. As much as we wanted her, we put aside our feelings and decided to interrupt the pregnancy. I went through eighteen hours of labor, and she was born at 1:52 A.M. on a Thursday morning. She was perfect and beautiful. We held her and looked at her and wished she could stay with us. Our arms hurt to hold her again. Although she was perfect to us, she had overlapping fingers, clubfeet, low-set ears, and an elongated head. Her internal anomalies were numerous. She had large, bilateral choroid plexus cysts, small left heart, brain stem disorder, a hole in the main ventricle, and other conditions. It was amazing to us how much we loved this little girl. However, she would be in a better place than we were, and she would indeed be perfect and beautiful and healthy. We constantly tell ourselves this, although it does not make us feel any better yet. We want to have more children, but we don't think it will be the same. Most people think that your grief should be measured by the size of your baby, that we should think of it as a miscarriage and move on. These people are sorely mistaken. We cherish the memories we have of our daughter! We are sure the choice we made to see her, hold her, name her, have mementos of her, was the best thing we could have done to make sure she would never be replaced or forgotten! We look forward to our next pregnancy, but our hearts are sore from the loss of our sweet daughter!

Prayer and Hope

First, I offer prayers and blessings to all of you who have experienced the loss of a child. There is no darker or longer time in your life, but at the end of my story, I hope some of you will find a fraction of the joy that now abounds in my life. My son was born at 42 weeks. We had a troublefree pregnancy. He was our first child. He was perfect but for one small problem: he had a huge hole in his diaphragm. This is not deadly, we were told, but his abdominal organs, including a portion of his liver, had migrated to his chest cavity. Therefore, his lungs could never develop. We made the decision to have him transferred to a hospital an hour away so that surgery could be performed in an attempt to save his life. I arrived at the hospital shortly before he died. My husband swears he was waiting for me, because his vital signs (never good, but stable) dropped as soon as I arrived at the hospital. We talked with the neonatologist and asked him the prognosis. He responded, head bowed and voice soft, "We do not aggressively resuscitate an infant in this condition." What to do? I wanted to remove the life support. Surprisingly, I did not need time to think about this. Enough is enough. It was so hard to look my husband in the eye and tell him I wanted to let his firstborn son go. But when I did look at him, I saw the same love and pain struggle. We bathed our son, removed all the tubes, the monitors, and finally the respirator. I held him in my arms for the first and last time. What a bittersweet memory. He lived only eighteen hours. It is our belief that God had a small soul who needed a lifetime of love in a very short period of time, and we were there to give it.

At our baby's memorial service, we decided to try for another baby as soon as medically possible. What surprised us both was the year it took my body to be ready. Six infertility doctors, two surgeries, drugs, and sperm counts later, we were blessed with another son. We were told to come back when we were ready to conceive again. Well, they have turned me on, and can't turn me off! We now have three healthy boys, ages six, four, and two. A very wise woman said to me once, "If God did not want you to have children, he would take away your desire for children. It is just in his time and his way." Infertility treatments, adoption, or reaching troubled kids. All kids are a gift. No matter how long you have them with you on earth, you will always carry the gift in your heart. It will strengthen you, define your future decisions, and, if you allow it, bathe you in a warmth like no other.

Anna

We just gave birth to our beautiful daughter Anna. She lived fifteen hours, and they were the most wonderful in my life. She had Potter's Syndrome and her kidneys shrank to nothing. We knew that she had just a slim chance of coming out with adequate lung development. My amniotic fluid was found to be low at 18 weeks and just went down from there. I went into labor at 35.5 weeks. We had planned a C-section to give her every chance we could. I guess it was not enough. I remember lying there, unable to see over the screen and asking my husband over and over if he could see her yet. I remember hearing a little cry—the only sound that I would ever hear her make. I thought that meant she had good lungs. I was so happy for those few minutes. I knew that her kidneys were bad, but we were so prepared to go the long haul! We were ready for peritoneal dialysis and then a kidney transplant. I would not give up on her. They took me into the NICU on a gurney and let me see her. Soon I got up and, in a wheelchair, spent the rest of her life in the NICU touching her. They finally told me her vital signs were dipping down and that I should hold her, perhaps for the last time. My husband got a children's book and read to her. Her vital signs improved for a while at the sound of his voice. We had been reading to her in my stomach during the whole pregnancy, and I pray that she was comforted in the end by his voice. Her hair was so soft.

My Boy

I write this message twenty-seven days after the loss of my son. Everyone says it gets better. It does, really. I haven't cried in days, and I can even laugh and smile. (Sometimes I feel guilty when I do, though. How can I smile so soon after having lost my baby?) I have returned to work and to life in general. The distraction of doing everyday things helps, although it is so difficult to go back to having a "normal" life. My husband summed it up best by saying, "How can our lives change so much, but still change so little?"

Time is creeping by. I remember how it seemed to fly by during my pregnancy. I still have two months to wait before we can try again. Then nine more months before we can bring home a baby. I am frustrated. I know how many weeks pregnant I should be: 25 weeks. I obviously canceled the prenatal visit I had scheduled for today. I think I have started to move into the "anger" phase of grieving. I'm not mad at anyone in particular, just mad at the world for being so cruel. Although I know I'll never have the answers, I can't help asking Why us? Why did my perfect little boy have to die?

I have learned how to walk down the baby aisle in the grocery store. I can't look at the products on the shelves, but it's a start. I can look at pregnant women, but I can't smile at them yet. I can see babies, but I can't touch them yet. I have stopped envisioning a car seat in the rearview mirror. I am learning that my hand doesn't belong on my stomach. I have stopped calling my husband "Dad" and my mom "Grandma." I have quit planning for maternity leave. I still pass off wanting chocolate as a "craving," though! This is the hardest time of my life, but I'm making it through with the help of a loving husband and the support of friends and family.

Sharing

I think I am ready to share now—I need to share. When I felt the baby move—oh, it was so amazing, like a total flop in my tummy. It had finally happened! I felt I was entering a new phase of my pregnancy. On July 10 I went to see my doctor for my four-month checkup. I was 17 weeks' pregnant and feeling so good. I wore a cute little dress and felt so smug, and I was delighted with my new tummy and my healthy little baby. It was all about to go very wrong. The baby had no heartbeat . . . it was not moving.

My husband and I spent the weekend in each other's arms, crying, talking about what we wanted to happen with the birth of our first child who had died. Would we see it? What would it look like? Would this hurt physically? How much? My husband, a physician, later told me he was totally unprepared for the next two days.

Sunday night we went to the hospital and they put these sponges in my cervix that would dilate overnight so I could be induced Monday morning. The pain was searing as they were put in, but it was nothing compared to the pain I experienced as I lay on the bed in the antenatal ward, listening to the fetal heart monitors in the next room. Luckily I did not have to spend the night with all the healthy pregnant women waiting to give birth. They sent me home to a sleepless night with horrible cramping.

Monday we arrived at the hospital at 7 A.M. (my mom arrived shortly after). Soon my doctor came in to take out the sponges and put prostaglandin in my cervix that would induce me. The perinatal crisis worker came to see us and basically informed us that this was going to be a full labor, an average of ten to twelve hours. How would I do this? Then I felt something coming out of me—my water had broken. I felt so sad, so cheated—my first experience with any of this, and it was so dreadfully wrong.

At 5:25 in the evening, our first baby was born. I sit here and I can still feel her coming out, the umbilical cord hanging outside of me. We held the baby and cried for what should have been. She was perfectly formed, like a tiny doll. I felt so calm, so proud of this little baby, and yet so awful. The hospital gave me a mahogany box with pictures of the baby, a blanket they wrapped her in, her footprints, the hospital bracelets we would have worn, and a crib card. These mementos are so dear to me now when I sit and wonder if this really happened.

Now I sit here a childless mother. I had a baby. I lactated, but no one knows this. In the last week two friends have had their first babies, I feel so much pain and anger toward them. Why me? One minute I think I am fine, and the next minute I am a total wreck. I am so tired all the time. I have lost my innocence, my faith in life. Only a miracle will bring it back.

My Son

In June 1995, we found out we were pregnant after a heartbreaking early miscarriage nine months before. We were so scared, but the pregnancy went very well. Because of the miscarriage and the insensitive care we received at the hospital, we had decided to have this second baby at home, barring any complications. It went beautifully, and on March 19, 1996, I had an 8-pound, 4-ounce, baby boy at 41 weeks after an easy labor. His Apgar score was low at first, but soon he was doing fine. All went well until early morning of the third day, when he became fussy and refused to nurse. He began vomiting, and I struggled with feeling like a paranoid first-time mother and panicking. I made an appointment with our pediatrician for 8:30 that morning. By the time the doctor saw him, he was gasping for breath and was dusky colored. The doctor had the baby transferred via ambulance to the PICU at the nearest hospital. At the hospital, we were told that he had hypoplastic left heart syndrome and that he needed surgery or a heart transplant to survive the following weeks. Babies have an uphill battle with this type of heart defect. The cardiologist also gave us the option to medicate him to make him more comfortable and let him die naturally. We couldn't believe what he was saying. We went from what we considered the ideal birth situation to facing the death of our dear baby. For six days, while they were getting him stabilized, we struggled with what to do, and finally agreed to let the doctors try the surgery. Miles only had a 50–50 chance of making it, but we had to go with the choice that we could live with for the rest of our lives. I already felt so bad for not seeing the signs of his illness earlier and taking him to the hospital sooner, so he wouldn't have had to suffer. I couldn't take from him the only chance he had. He didn't survive the surgery, which they performed on the eighth day of his life. We were numb. The PICU nurse asked if we wanted to see his body, but I felt like we had already had several days of very special bonding, so I refused. I didn't want to see the wound on his chest, or for that to be my last memory of him. I don't regret that to this day. I feel so fortunate to have been able to nurse him and hold him in our bed at home for two and a half days.

The past year has been rocky. We have lost several friends because they are having children, and the loss of our son probably threatens their rose-colored picture of the way things are supposed to be. I have my son's ashes at home and still cannot bear to part with them. Maybe I never will. I feel lucky that my relationship with my husband has stayed strong throughout this tragedy. We had another early miscarriage three months after Miles's death, which was very hard to take. I think I lost the last shred of my innocence and hopeful assumptions about childbearing after that miscarriage. We are now 24 weeks' pregnant and have had a good result with a fetal echocardiogram that was done at 20 weeks. But I still can't imagine having a baby to keep when this is over in July. We found out it is another boy, and he kicks vigorously every day. But I know now how fragile a baby's life is, and I can't let myself fully enjoy the experience.

Twins

I was diagnosed with Twin-to-Twin Transfusion Syndrome at 19 weeks and found out that I had been in premature labor for the past month or two. My identical twin sons were sharing a single placenta. One son was classified as the stuck twin; he was getting very little of the nutrients from the placenta, and my other son was getting almost all of it. The second son had an excessive amount of amniotic fluid, and the first had so little that he could barely move. I was put on strict bed rest and given Terbutaline and Magnesium Sulfate to stop labor.

At 27 weeks, I told the nurses that one son wasn't acting right. They said I was an overworried mother, even though my son's heartbeat was faint. I was brought to ultrasound an hour later, at 1:00 P.M., and my son was dead. The staff then took me to the maternity floor and stopped my gurney next to a mother and her newborn baby, and left me there with this child crying in my ear. My heart was broken, my dreams were shattered, and all I could think about was my son who was alive and the one who wasn't. It wasn't fair to him or to me that he would have to go through life without his brother.

After a week and a half I told the doctors I needed to go home and recover with my family. They told me I could have my twins anytime.

I went into labor, and my first son weighed 3 pounds, 15 ounces. My second son was stillborn shortly thereafter, and weighed 2 pounds, 14 ounces. My first son was rushed off to NICU; they tossed my stillborn son into a cold metal basin and carried him away. They brought him back an hour later, dressed in one of the matching outfits I had bought for my boys. He was resting in a wicker basket made for dolls. I never lifted him out of the basket for fear that he would break. He was so perfect in every way. I counted his toes and undressed him to see everything about him. His life may have been over, but his love and charm will always remain.

My dead son gave his life so that his brother could live. To me he will always be my hero. I have ultrasound videos of my sons playing together and I have a picture of my dead son smiling at me. These are the only live memories I have of my dead son, and they are the most treasured memories of my life. I know that Christian is a part of his brother and always will be, and for that I am truly thankful.

Three

My husband and I have tried for over four years to have a baby. My first pregnancy ended in miscarriage at 6 weeks' gestation. We never saw the sac on the ultrasound, only the spot where it had been after the miscarriage started. It was doomed from the start; my progesterone was low and the HCG numbers rose erratically. We waited a few months and then tried intrauterine inseminations again. On our third wedding anniversary, we found out that we were pregnant again. My HCG numbers quadrupled within forty-eight hours. On February 28, I had some slight spotting and went in for an ultrasound. We found two sacs. We were having twins. Things seemed fine for a few weeks, but then I passed a blood clot. We went to the doctor and he was able to find one heartbeat; the other one was still a bit small. I stayed home and in bed. One week later, I woke up and felt a "pop," then began to hemorrhage. I passed one of the twins at home. I was rushed to the doctor. My bleeding became worse, and soon I was passing clots the size of baseballs. We were not able to determine if the other baby had a heartbeat, but I was bleeding to death. (I lost half my blood supply in a few hours.) They did a D&C, and once again I went home, crushed.

My grief was so deep that I could only think about getting pregnant again. Two months later, I had another insemination, against my husband's better judgment. I got a positive pregnancy test twelve days after the insemination. The next day I went to the doctor. My HCG numbers were very high, considering I was five days away from being supposed to have my period. My back ached horribly, and I began to have sciatic nerve pain. The next week, after my HCG numbers had risen exponentially, I had an ultrasound and found that we were having quads! Two days later I had some spotting, so I went back to the doctor. One of the sacs had stopped developing and was going to reabsorb. It looked like my triplets were there to stay. On the first day of my sixth week, I had a routine ultrasound and found all three heartbeats! But as I left the office, I felt something was wrong. I could not stop crying. As I went home to change for work, I started to bleed. Soon I was passing clots. I rushed back to the doctor. All three were still there and my cervix was closed. She put me on bed rest. For the next six weeks I had huge bleeding episodes and passed big clots. Each time I went in, they cleaned me up, watched me for a while, and then sent me home. The babies were fine. I had a cervical cerclage in my twelfth week, since my cervix seemed short and one of the babies was lying right over it. That baby (I later found out) was the source of all my bleeding, coming from her placenta. At my thirteenth week I went back to work. Six hours into my first day I had another massive bleeding episode. This time, with my cervix tied shut, the clots pressed down and strained to get through. I was in excruciating pain. I was taken off the blood thinners I had been on to suppress my antibody problems that may have caused my two previous miscarriages. I stayed home in bed.

At the 19-week ultrasound we found that we were carrying two girls and a boy (just as we had thought). We also found out that I was funneling—my cervix was trying to open up and my uterus was ballooning out at the bottom. The baby over my cervix (we named her Rebecca Nicole) had changed position. She was engaged, her little head crammed against the cervix. I was sent home with some indocin and ordered to stay off my feet at all costs. A week later, I woke up at 3 A.M. to use the bathroom. I noticed a lot of mucus. I began to have contractions that morning, They were calmed somewhat by the Indocin®. By that evening the contractions had become painful. I went to the hospital at 8:30 and found that I was dilated 3 centimeters with the cerclage still in. My doctor removed the cerclage and I was put into bed with the bed tilted backward. It was certain that Rebecca would come. The doctor told me that if they all came that day, they would have no hope for survival. I stayed awake all night, feeling them kick and bargaining with God. By dawn I knew they would all be born.

The first daughter was born. She was so perfect, but very red and very small. She lived for about forty-five minutes. Then my second daughter was born. She was the smallest, but still so beautiful. She held on to life for thirty minutes. By this time I was bleeding heavily, having passed neither placenta. The doctor felt the last sac coming down slowly. She put me on pitocin to induce his birth; otherwise, she would have to operate, because I was losing so much blood. At 1:23 P.M. my son was born. He was far bigger than his sisters, and he lived for about an hour. My angels were so beautiful; I was overjoyed that I was able to hold my children and so devastated that they had died.

It has been a long, hard road for me and my husband. He seems better than I am, but he has never gone to see their grave (the hospital cremated them and put their ashes in a stone monument at a cemetery along with the ashes of other babies who died there that year). We will try again, but this time we want to be more financially prepared. My husband wants to have six months' worth of expenses in the bank so we won't have to worry, as I am sure I will be on bed rest again. My doctor has told me that with my weak cervix I cannot carry more than twins, and we cannot afford IVF. We have decided that if I get pregnant with higher-order multiples again, we will not reduce; we will take it as far as we can. I still have nightmares and I still cry when I see other pregnant women or other babies. But it will happen. Someday we will have a child to raise.

My Story

My story begins with the arrival of my first daughter, Angela Katherine, on October 12, 1981. After seven hours in labor and an epidural, I underwent an emergency cesarean under general anesthetic. It took some time to recover from the experience, both physically and mentally, but I was thankful to have a healthy daughter and have been grateful ever since that the doctors had the foresight to undertake the operation to save both my daughter's life and my own. It is only now, with a lot of hindsight, that I realize how lucky I was to come home after ten days with my baby girl in my arms.

On May 4, 1985, I gave birth to my second daughter, Alison Hannah, after nine and a half hours' labor with an epidural that worked on only one side and a vaginal delivery. I was on a high almost immediately following her birth, having thought a vaginal delivery would not be possible following the cesarean. Unfortunately, Alison went into distress during labor and swallowed and inhaled meconium. There was little that could be done once her lungs were filled. All we could do was pray that she would pull through and come home to meet her big sister.

Sadly, after twenty-seven hours, Alison's fight for life was over. She died in my arms on May 5, 1985, a day I will never forget as long as I live. There are no words to explain how I felt deep inside at letting go of the child I had longed to get pregnant with. I had enjoyed a textbook pregnancy, planning for the future. My life came to a standstill as I tried hard to retain some normality for the sake of my older daughter. Angela had so wanted a sister. She kept saying she wanted a friend, not a brother.

We buried Alison at a local cemetery where other members of my family are resting. We had a nice funeral for her and involved Angela in everything. How she coped with it all made me feel so proud. If only adults could behave in the way Angela did. So innocent and unaffected by the attitude of older people who wanted me to leave her behind as we laid her sister to rest. I feel it made a difference in her life, and she still remembers Alison with affection and love. We take flowers for Alison on her birthday and Christmas and any other time I feel I need to have time alone to share with her quietly. I am lucky that I have photographs taken of Alison, since the last thing I was thinking of was a camera. Without the photographs, I probably would have forgotten with the passing of the years what my little girl looked like. How lucky I was that the nursing staff was so thoughtful!

I was fortunate to have an understanding doctor who never tired of my asking to look at the record of Alison's birth and death. I stayed in touch for a long time with the student midwife whose first delivery was Alison. My family were and always have been very supportive; friends, too, have been a valuable help in my grieving process. The grief has never stopped; the memories are still as fresh today. I just have to learn to live with my feelings, because I know I can't change what happened. I'm grateful for the experience of having two little girls. I had a very different birth experience with each of them, and I am thankful I was able to experience a vaginal delivery, which at one time was thought to be only a desire after a cesarean. Sadly, I may never be able to experience it again because of medical problems, but I have the satisfaction of having brought my daughters into the world, albeit in very different ways.

I have known the desperation of wanting to be pregnant. I have carried my children and seen them arrive in this world. I am one of the lucky ones. After a lot of soul searching, I decided the time was right to try for another child. I had divorced and am now with my new husband, who has been very supportive in my darkest moments. He has been my rock when things have gotten just a little too hard to bear. Angela sees him as her father.

It took only a very short time to conceive, and our elation was obvious. We told only close family and friends, wanting to wait until we had reached 12 weeks just to be on the safe side. Not for a moment did we think anything would go wrong; we just wanted to be cautious.

On December 17, 1996, I had an appointment with the hospital consultant. We discussed the birth, which would undoubtedly be an elective cesarean, but he told me not to worry about it as I was only ten weeks and there was plenty of time to organize things. I asked if I could have a scan just to put my mind at rest, since I had been feeling slightly different during that day. I was sent for a scan within minutes, just to confirm everything was all right.

As my husband, my sister, and I sat in the scan waiting room, I felt as if I was bleeding. I went to the ladies room to check, and I was. Andrew tried to reassure me that everything was going to be fine, but I knew in my heart that things were not as they should be. As I lay on the bed in the scan room, the operator took what seemed like an age to find our baby. Then the fatal words came: "I'm sorry, but I can't seem to find a fetus; the sac appears to be empty." I knew then that it was all over and that our plans for the future would have to be adjusted. I had so desperately wanted this baby, as I had my other two children. The maternal instinct was very strong and couldn't be erased. I was only 10 weeks' pregnant, but I was carrying a child inside of me. I had lost again, and no one seemed able to console me. I still cry and wonder what might have been, but now feel as if things are getting a little easier to bear. I have tried so hard to put thoughts of babies out of my mind, but I am unable to do this. It's at the forefront of my mind all the time, and until I can bring Andrew's baby home, a sister or brother for Angela, I will not feel totally at peace within myself.

I used to think that miscarriage was something that happened to other people, not to me. I was the one it wouldn't happen to. How wrong I was. My sister has had three miscarriages and each time has been devastated by the pain of it all. She used to say it was worse for me losing Alison because I had gone to full term. But now, having experienced a miscarriage myself, I can say in all honesty that the pain was just as acute, though a little different. Our grief cannot be measured on a scale of 1–10. We can grieve for what we have never had as well as for what we have had and lost.

As far as I am concerned, I have had three children, of which I am very proud. The excitement of being pregnant and anticipating the arrival of a new life in the world is something that cannot be explained. I am deeply grateful for being able to live the excitement; some are not so lucky. I cannot imagine what my life would have been like had I not been able to be pregnant at all. I suppose I would have coped, as I have coped with the loss of two of my children. My sister has never pursued things with the medical profession, and may never have the joy of giving birth to her own child.

Loss and grief are very personal emotions. You cannot fully explain to someone exactly how you feel. You can only hope that someone has the compassion to try and understand. Others who have been in a similar position will know the depth of your grief, but your own loss is very personal to you. Some people feel unable to discuss the matter with you, because they do not fully understand your grief and fear hurting your feelings. People can seem very cruel at times, but only because they do not want to bring up something that they feel may hurt you.

Following Alison's death I was treated very well by the hospital staff. After my miscarriage, I was admitted for a D&C at the hospital, then came home. I received little support at all, and it hurt. Only with time have I learned to come to terms with things, and felt strong enough to try and do something positive out of my grief. I have arranged to attend a local miscarriage support group in the near future and have already joined the Miscarriage Association. I have often said I would love to write a book, so this may be a starting point for me. I don't know all the answers. I am living my own private grief, but maybe in some small way I can help others who have had the trauma of loss.

We all came from our mothers. We must continue the search for answers to all the questions we have. Why do so many women miscarry? What, if anything, can be done to prevent it or reduce the risk? Or is it really just nature's way, an explanation we must accept from people who do not fully understand what we have endured? Thankfully, since I lost Alison I have never heard of any other children dying from the same fate. So maybe things have improved greatly. In the early 1980s I would never have dreamed that so much could have happened to me. I will never know where I've found my strength. I sit with the photographs of Alison and cry. I keep her memory alive by talking about her, so that people know of her existence. Angela still recalls the memory of her baby sister and still hopes to be blessed one more time. I hope I can give her the chance again to have a sister or brother before she grows up too much and loses interest. I want to give Andrew a child of his own and see the joy it will bring into his life. Most of all, I want to be a mother. Bake bread, sing, do all the things I wanted to do, but work got in the way.

I have seemed to throw myself deeply into my work. It has been an escape for me, something I have a reasonable amount of control over. Now the time has come to put things into perspective and to realize that we pass this way only once. There are things in life all people want, and I am determined to get some of what I want and need. If it doesn't happen, I'll know there was a reason for it, just as there were reasons for losing Alison and my 10 weeks' pregnancy.

Our Baby Girl

On December 27, I was told that my baby had spina bifida and hydro-cephalus. I was 21 weeks' pregnant. My husband is in the Air Force, and the military hospital wouldn't do an ultrasound, so my mother paid for me to have one done as a Christmas present. Mom is a nurse, and she felt at least one ultrasound was necessary. I really took the health of the baby for granted. We were going for the ultrasound for the fun of it, to find out if it was a girl or a boy. How trivial that was! Mom, Dad, and my husband were all in the room when we found out our baby had spina bifida. Dad turned his head to the wall so I wouldn't see his tears. It was so horrible. I didn't know what spina bifida meant, but I know Mom did. Our baby girl had paralyzed legs, clubfoot, and a very large cyst on her back that was obvious on the ultrasound. It appeared to be a third of the size of her body. I never realized that the reason I had barely felt her move until the last week was because her legs were paralyzed. The doctor who did the ultrasound was a very wonderful woman. She told me she was sorry, and she even cried with us. She said it would take some soul searching to decide what we would do. Outside influences on our decision were to be avoided, since my hus-band and I would be the ones to live with whatever we decided. That was the best advice we got.

The doctor gave us the name of a neurosurgeon who would talk to us about his experiences with children with spina bifida and the name of a doctor who could do a genetic termination if that was what we decided. After the neurosurgeon had reviewed the ultrasound tape, he couldn't tell us much. I wanted someone to tell me that my daughter would be OK, other than having to be in a wheelchair. A wheelchair and paralysis could be OK; mental retardation and brain shunts were another issue. The neu-rosurgeon told us hydrocephalus of her degree at 21 weeks was not a pos-itive indication. No one could predict her fate, so, unfortunately, this decision was placed on our shoulders. It was very sad. I don't think my heart or soul has ever felt so heavy. I had just begun to feel her move Christmas Eve. It was her hands moving. It is almost as if it were her way of letting me know she was real, her way of communicating with me for the first and last time. She gave me that gift to remember her by. My mother and husband felt her move ever so slightly.

When my husband and I decided to have the termination, it was unbear-able. We wanted her so badly, but the thought of placing a shunt in her brain for hydrocephalus and other numerous intrusions made this the right thing for her and for us. I cried and cried when I felt her move the night before the termination. My husband hugged my belly and cried. It's hard to admit, but I hoped the drugs they gave me would cause her to sleep so

I wouldn't feel her move. It was so heart-wrenching to feel her move inside me. The next day at the clinic, I went into the bathroom so I could tell my daughter good-bye in private. I couldn't even look at myself in the mirror, because it made it more real.

Today, I have a bit more peace about her death. I know she is safe now in the arms of an angel, but I miss her. I know that the termination was a horrible choice to have to make, but we did the best we could with the knowledge we had. At this moment I am disappointed that all of the medical advances we have today lay these kinds of issues in the hands of women instead of letting things take their natural course. On the other hand, I am grateful to have had the chance to meet my baby via ultrasound. I watch it alone sometimes. My husband won't watch it. Somehow all of this will make sense someday. For now we are still healing and missing her.

My Son

In 1992 I found out at about 20 weeks of pregnancy that my baby was anencephalic. I was told that this was always fatal and that I should terminate the pregnancy as soon as possible. It was not an easy decision, but I wanted this baby for as long as I could have him. I decided to carry him to term. It was a long five months of waiting and crying. I can't honestly say there was a lot of hoping. I knew that he wasn't going to live. They told me he most likely would not live through birth. I had great support from my doctor, which helped. Most everyone else just chose to pretend I was no longer pregnant. My son was born by C-section. He did live through birth and then for five days. He was a beautiful baby, at least in my eyes. We were able to bring him home from the hospital, and he spent a day with us there before he died on December 21, 1992. We buried our son on Christmas Eve. I have never regretted my decision to continue my pregnancy. It was a decision made for a lot of reasons. Mostly, I think because I felt he was safe there. No one could take him away when he was still inside of me. I wanted him for as long as I could have him. There is a saying that goes "We hold our children's hands for a while; their hearts, forever." I truly believe this. We don't know how much time we have with our children. It is time to be cherished and enjoyed. I had time with my son, nine months of pregnancy and five precious days of life. I have since had another child, another boy. I am also blessed to have had my older son to help get me through the pain and loneliness of losing my son. I will always be thankful for his gift, and I will forever miss him and wish we had him longer.

My Son

I have a hard time telling this story. I know that everyone else does, too, but that doesn't make it easier. After six months of a very complicated pregnancy, my son died in utero. I tried so hard to do everything right, and it wasn't enough. It was one of the first times in my life I could not make something happen by sheer force of will. I was only twenty-one, married three weeks, when we found out I was pregnant. We were young, scared, and poor, but have such loving and supportive families that we finally decided to go ahead with the pregnancy. It never occurred to me that something could go wrong. I had no risk factors, didn't smoke, didn't drink, and yet something was wrong with the implantation in my uterus that stunted and eventually ended my baby's life. The experiences I had with the doctors were awful. They were condescending, accusatory; they acted as if they couldn't understand why I couldn't "get with the program" and accept what was happening. They kept talking about next time, but I was still thinking about this time. I had already felt him move, I had seen him kick and hiccup on the ultrasound. My husband told me that during my amniocentesis the baby turned and moved toward the needle when it went into the sac. I already had a happy, inquisitive little soul bouncing around in there. How was I supposed to pick up and go on? In the end, I did find a wonderful doctor who tried very hard to save the pregnancy, but my son died at the beginning of his 26th week. I went into labor later that day and got to see my beautiful, beautiful son. I am so grateful that I had the chance to see, hold, and name my child. I have an enormous debt of gratitude to the nurses who helped me that day, especially the one who broke the sac and cleaned his tiny body, wrapped him in a blanket, and took pictures of him. At the time I could not appreciate it, but now it gives me great comfort that she was so strong and kind. My son was so perfect, the neatest blend of my husband and my father—my two favorite men. His tiny blue eyes were open and he looked peaceful and wise, as if his soul had drifted in and out of the womb noiselessly. Seeing his face, I knew he would have been just like my husband: kind, calm, wise, and good. I miss him so much.

Comfort and Peace

When we lost our first baby, we were utterly crushed to find out that he had died four days or so previously. I seemed to know this at some level, because I was strangely frightened of visiting our doctor for the first ultrasound, while my husband was so excited about it. The last few days we have gone from hope and joy to despair, and I am lucky to have such a loving and supportive partner who has gone through agony with me during this heartbreaking time. We did something that brought us comfort and peace—we went down to the sea with flowers and incense. We found some driftwood in the shape of a little boat and placed our offering inside it with a letter of love and farewell to our baby. We said some special words, read our letter, and burned our incense, then set our little boat into the turning tide—which is the metaphor for all of life. The passing of someone so dear and special should not go unnoticed. No one else knows of our loss, but this doesn't matter now, because we were lent our child only briefly, and with our farewell we take him back into ourselves for all time. I thought others might like to know that what seemed too hard to do a few days ago, actually helped us immeasurably at a terrible time. It was a release for all three of us, yet also a coming together. There need be no parting of this union ever again.

We buried our son at a very nice place at the cemetery that is only for children, so now he's got some friends, I hope. The whole summer was a long, long mourning period. I was always crying or at least felt very sad. I thought that I was the one to blame. Maybe I did something wrong that caused his death. The most difficult part has been to explain everything to our daughter, but now I think she has understood everything that she can. Even if she is only three years old, she sometimes surprises me by knowing a lot of things I didn't think she would know. Sometimes she says to me, "Mum, can't we go and visit my brother today?" Things like that make me warm in my heart. We have been talking very much about the loss in the family. A lot of our friends have disappeared. They don't know what to say, or say the wrong things and are afraid to make contact with us again.

When I read all the stories about all the pain and heartache that are felt worldwide, it saddens me, but in a way it comforts me; I am not alone. Strangers we may be, yet we are connected by a common thread; the loss of a child makes us all soul mates. When our son was born, I thought I had his whole life to hold him. Foolish what we think! In my case a whole lifetime lasted only three days. When our son died, our fairytale turned into a nightmare. I did not care about anything. My husband, despite his pain, pulled me back from the brink of insanity, and my family held me together. If ever a viewing and a funeral could be beautiful, his were. We picked two songs to be played at the cemetery, and then we released three blue balloons into the sky. It was as if an angel came right out of the sky and took the balloons with invisible hands into the heavens. It's been almost a year, and the pain is still as strong. Zachary is a part of my life forever. He lives in my heart, and as his gravestone says, "We will hold you in heaven."

Unending Love

It's hard not to feel alone and that no one understands when you are experiencing a loss. My husband and I have lost three pregnancies in the last two years. All first trimester—no heartbeat and blighted ovum. I could probably write for hours about the emotional drain and depression I have felt. I am certainly not the same person I was two years ago, and the sad part is, my family and friends notice, too—I thought I was hiding it better. If I hadn't had the unending love and support of my husband, I would probably be a mental vegetable by now. We waited to start a family—I am thirty-three—because I loved my work and was determined to build a successful career. Now I sit here at work and I don't feel like doing a thing. My work used to be my life; now I couldn't care less. The hardest part is watching my friends and family members have successful pregnancies, and watching the children at church—even going to church. It's hard to believe in a God who would put you through this much agony.

It's been almost a year since the birth and death of our beautiful daughter. Like everyone else's stories, ours started the same way. Everything seemed to be fine until an ultrasound revealed some growth abnormalities. I had made up my mind that I could deal with a child with severe abnormalities, but my daughter had lethal anomalies and would die at birth. I carried her until my 34th week, when went into labor. Throughout my long labor her heartbeat was strong, and I prayed that was a sign things were not as grave as I had been told. At 7:42 P.M. she was born into this world. At 7:43 she left it. I was devastated. My sweet little baby girl, the little girl I had dreamed of having my entire life, was taken from me as quickly as she was given to me. We kept her with us until almost midnight. We held her and kissed her and gave her as much love as we could during that short period of time. I thought I would die when my husband carried her out of the room to give her to the funeral home. I have a lot of pictures of her, but sometimes I ache from wanting to feel her. We had a funeral and she's buried in our family plot. I visit her often. For Christmas this year I put a little Christmas tree up at her grave. I miss her. The pain has come back greatly since I also suffered a miscarriage in my 7th week within the year. I've lost two babies in one year. Do I dare to try again?

I feel like I have these different voices in my head with conflicting opinions. I hear the one strongly that is saying, "What if something awful happens again? Maybe you should just quit while you're ahead." I believe the desire for another baby is stronger than this voice. This has been a terrible blow to our family. I find myself struggling to find solid ground, a new belief system, because the old one didn't include a "nice" family like ours losing a newborn baby. Someone at a hospice bereavement support group (open to anyone) told me that grief is a very powerful thing. I liked that description, because it doesn't tell you how you should do it or when, or how you should feel. This experience has changed me like an earthquake that has ripped through all of our lives. Perhaps ultimately the effects can be good. I would like her little life to have brought good somehow.

My Story

I saw you on the monitor today. For the last sixteen weeks I've been trying to pretend you're not there. Not an easy task when I'm throwing up everything nightly, crying at the drop of a hat, especially when those sappy commercials come on, and all the hormonal changes that a body goes through when it's creating a new life. As impossible as it is, I've tried to keep you out of my thoughts, out of my prayers, out of my heart.

It's not that I don't want to love you, but please try to understand that after losing four others, I'm hoping that if I ignore your very existence, and I lose you, too, the wound to my heart won't go as deep. Maybe this time it won't hurt so much. But here you are on the ultrasound screen, ruining all my well laid plans. I try to see you as the world does: to them you're only a fetus, just a blur on the screen. If I don't listen, I won't hear the beat of your heart. If I keep my eyes from focusing, I can't make out your face, your hands, your tiny feet. The doctor leaves the room. I try to turn away. I can't. Instead, I reach out and trace your image in front of me. From the bottom of my soul my heart cries out to you, speaking the feelings I've tried so hard to repress. "Please fight, little one. Please hold on. I do want you, I do love you. Please fight." Hard as I try, I can't stop the hope and joy I feel. Maybe this time. Your heartbeat is so strong, everything seems fine. Maybe I can let you in.

It's been four days since I've seen you. It's 1:00 A.M. Something has wakened me. I lie in bed for a few moments, wondering what it might be. Then the feeling comes. Something isn't right. The tears begin to fall. "No," I tell myself, "I'm just being paranoid, everything is fine." But the tears won't stop. I slip out of bed and go downstairs. I don't want to wake your father.

You're gone. I know it somehow; and yet I begin to pray in spite of that knowledge, willing not to believe it. There's no proof you're gone, right? I pray and pray, pleading with Heavenly Father to give me peace, to let me know that everything is fine. The tears begin to fall faster as the confirmation won't come. Hours later, when the tears won't come anymore, I return to bed, exhausted. Your father asks, "What's wrong?" He's come to trust my feelings. He knows now, as do I, that you're gone. We hold each other and cry. But still, deep down inside, I am hoping against hope that I am wrong.

Once again I am seeing you on the monitor. Straining my ears to hear your heartbeat again, not wanting to blink as I stare at the screen, fearing I might miss a slight movement that would prove my worries wrong. The doctor turns off the screen. "I just don't understand it," he says, "everything was just fine the other day." My mind screams, "Try again, turn the monitor back on. Maybe you're sleeping, maybe we didn't wait long enough." Sobs shake my body. I try to keep you safe by wrapping my arms around my body. Maybe if I hold tight enough, you'll be okay.

I know the next steps well. The hospital, the nurses, the doctors, all the preparations for removing you from my body. As I watch the hospital staff move around me, a silent war rages in my mind. What if they're wrong? What if they are planning to take you from me, and you're still alive? Should I ask them to try again? The fight continues even as they wheel me into surgery. My fears are never voiced as I fall into deep sleep. I awaken; you're gone. They tell me you weren't really real. This is for the best. Maybe you weren't forming right. It's much easier to lose you now than later. I never really knew you. I know they're trying to help. And I try to believe what they say. But if you were so unreal, then why does it seem I can smell your sweet soft skin? Feel your downy head on my cheek? If you weren't real, why is my heart breaking in two?

I don't know if I will ever find the words to explain the void I feel now that you're gone. How I long to touch your tiny fingers, to count each little toe. To hold your warm body next to mine. My arms ache from not holding you. They say that time heals all wounds. I know this is true. You'll be forgotten quickly by the world. They never saw you on the screen as I did. They never heard your heart beat with life. I'm not sure what you were to them. But you were my hopes and dreams, you were my future, and you will not be forgotten by me.

Precious Life

Through all the pain I have experienced, there has always been hope. I never really gave up hoping that there would be more joy in my life, though at times I struggled to believe I would ever feel the joy of holding another child of my own in my arms again. The grieving process is ongoing, and there will never be an end to the pain I feel from losing my children. I still ache and cry regularly for my daughter and have found it very difficult to accept her death, even after thirteen years.

How precious and fragile life is. Something I've come to appreciate much more since my son arrived into the world. I hold him close and shed a tear sometimes for what might have been with my daughter and my baby I miscarried. If not for them, I wouldn't have this lively, energetic, happy, bouncing baby boy. What greater gift could I wish for? I am grateful that I had the chance to try again. That feeling I had when my son was lifted aloft by my physician, in the first seconds of his life outside of the womb, cannot be compared to any other feeling I have had before or will have again. Through my contact with the bereavement services, I am healing better than in the past. I was never offered any form of counseling back in 1985, and so a lot of what I felt back then, came back in my recent pregnancy. I have made several new contacts and am touched by the way others want to share their experiences with me and the way they let me share my babies with them. I've cried many a tear for others in their sorrow, and now I want to give something back to them.

Brief Thoughts

We are struggling with our loss and each day seems to be a battle. We are sure that in time this pain will get less.

I am still unable to talk to anyone without bursting into tears. It has helped to read others' stories. Reading the stories and poems has helped me not to feel I am the only one who is still hurting. My grief is real.

I know the empty feeling. It is especially frustrating that most people discount how it feels to lose a baby when you are pregnant. . . . It has been so much harder than I thought. Recently I have gotten the feeling that my friends don't understand why I am still not over this.

I feel like time has helped even though this will never go away. I miss her terribly but have learned to live with her in my heart instead of in my arms.

The sadness will always be there, but my life is full and happy. The loss of my child helped me appreciate all children more. The loss also gave me courage to face other difficult things. After all, if I survived the loss of my child, I can survive *anything*!

I felt so empty when we left the hospital, and so sad for my husband, who stood strong for me and tried to show everyone he was okay. I think that it is harder for the fathers, because at least for the first few months I had the chance to feel the life growing inside of me.

It seems that everyone around me has completely forgotten my baby girl! I was actually told that I should just forget her because she wasn't a baby and didn't matter. . . . I cannot do that. I am completely consumed with the thought of my baby girl.

I found that I was all the time battling between trying to maintain what is expected of me as an employee, a spouse, a breadwinner of the family, and so on, while at the same time trying to move on from the grief that was at times all I could take. It seems everyone tries to get you to move on and not think about it, not realizing that you really don't choose to be weighted down, it's just the way it is. Grief is both emotional and physical. And it takes time.

I find that there is no escaping the grief. . . . I have realized, however, how much I have changed my life (career decisions, housing, future dreams) because I've expected to be a mother. . . . Now I am dealing with the fact that it may not happen. I think about this often. Giving up on the dreams is like giving up hope that I will ever be a mother. Keeping the dreams alive means forcing myself to deal with the pain of the loss every single disappointing month.

CAREGIVERS' VIEWS

The difficulty that caregivers (e.g., physicians, nurses, medical students, social service workers, counselors, hospital and office personnel, and family members) have in dealing with parents who have lost pregnancies and newborn children is well documented. Recognizing their needs, I have asked several of my colleagues to contribute to this volume. Their doing so has led to an increased awareness of their feelings about this most difficult of situations.

A Caregiver's Story of Her Personal Pregnancy Loss In Memory of Our Son, Joseph Michael

Karen Aresco

It was Friday when I knew something was very wrong. Actually, not much had gone right in my pregnancy: bed rest, bleeding, hyperemesis. But this was different. I felt an overwhelming sense of doom. I couldn't explain it, but I knew. I tried to believe everyone I spoke with: that it would be OK as long as I kept doing what I was doing, which was really nothing, just lying in bed and obsessing about what my baby would look like, sound like, who he would grow up to be, and what he would do in his lifetime. But my thoughts and dreams were always interrupted by a sense of anxiety that something would go wrong.

On this particular morning, I felt an unusual flutter of activity. Then, as the day wore on, the movements decreased. By the time my husband came home, I was in full panic. I hadn't felt the baby move all afternoon. I knew there was a problem; my five years' experience as a labor and delivery nurse had taught me that. But as my husband tried to calm me and talk to my son through my stomach, he began to move. My fears were quieted for the time being.

On Saturday, I didn't feel much movement at all. On Sunday, nothing. It seemed odd,—and I still feel somewhat guilty over this—but as I called my doctor, a sense of calmness came over me, almost relief. I had spoken with him several times over the 27 weeks of my pregnancy, and daily for the last three days. This call was different. He tried to reassure me that it would probably be all right, and I believe he really thought it would be; but when I got to the office and walked into the ultrasound room, I had already accepted that my baby had died. The ultrasound confirmed it. My doctor did not have to say a word. I saw that there was no longer a heartbeat.

Telling my family was so very difficult. They had all taken shifts being with me over the last six and a half months. This was really more *our* baby than just mine. We had all invested so much in this baby. I felt so guilty, like I had let all of them down.

Arrangements were made and I went into the hospital, where the horror continued. The hardest thing was seeing the looks on the faces of my co-workers. They really were like family to me. No one knew what to say or do. I felt like it was my job to make it easier for them by being tough. And I tried, but the look in their eyes over the next few days is what I remember most. I became very ill, and ultimately ended up needing a cesarean section. I was hardly conscious when the decision was made, but I remember again feeling relief; it would finally be over.

I didn't awake for several hours after surgery. I am not surprised, really. I hadn't slept much over the last several days. I think my body had just given in to the exhaustion. I awoke to see my husband sitting next to me. He looked so sad, yet at the same time I could see the love and relief in his eyes. My mother was there, too. She looked so worried, as did my dad when he came in. I remember feeling bad that I had caused so much trouble and worry for everyone.

Once I had washed my face, I felt a little better and wanted to see my son. I can vaguely recall the details. My vision was still blurry, but I remember thinking he looked so much like my husband. I looked him over from head to toe. He looked perfect, and that is how I will always remember him. I handed him to my husband, closed my eyes, and went back to sleep. My coworkers took pictures, handprints, and footprints of our son and put them in a memory book for us. I treasure this book and look at it often. It helps me feel closer to my son.

I stayed in the hospital a little over a week while my body began to recover physically. My emotions, on the other hand, were on a roller coaster. I went from sad to angry to guilty and back and forth in a matter of seconds. I kept asking Why? Why did this happen? I did everything I was supposed to do, and still this happened. Why? There were no answers to my questions. Many of my coworkers, family, and friends came to see me and lend their support. For them, I am so grateful. They will never know how much I appreciated all that they did for me, especially when I was being difficult. You see, mostly I was angry, and I took out my anger on those closest to me. I wanted them to hurt as much as I did. In my own grief, I couldn't see the pain that they were in. I was angry at myself and my body. I felt like a failure. I felt like I must have done something to have caused this. I felt like less of a woman because I could not do this right.

The day I left the hospital, I felt like I was abandoning my child. Although he wasn't physically with me any longer, I had felt better knowing we were in the same building. It was so hard to leave him behind. I was glad to be home once I got there, but at the same time, the reminders of what might have been were so hard to deal with. The book of names by my bedside, magazines on raising children, the needlepoint picture I was working on for his room—all things that helped pass the time while I was on bed rest now were a sign of what never would be. The hardest thing was looking into what would have been our son's room. I just closed the door; I couldn't deal with that emotion yet. My arms felt empty. I was longing to hold my precious baby. I was so very sad and lonely.

My mother helped us with the planning of the services and the burial for our son. My mother and husband picked out his casket. I couldn't. My mother purchased an outfit for him to wear. I pinned the guardian angel on the clothes. It was a gift from a friend during my pregnancy, and it seemed only fitting that I give it to my son, since I viewed him now as my special angel. I also gave to my mother, to put into his a casket, a stuffed musical elephant, a gift from my sister. I used to play it to my son. I remember how he moved to the sound. My brother put into the casket his altar boy cross from when he was a child. My mom and I picked out flowers and made an arrangement for the top of his casket. It was a small graveside service in the cemetery down the road from our house. I chose this cemetery because I knew I would be spending a lot of time there and also because I felt better knowing that he was so close to home. I went to the cemetery almost daily. I sat at my son's grave and talked to him, told him how I was feeling. Sometimes, I just cried. I was still trying to find an answer to the question Why.

Over the next several months, I tried to process all of what had happened. I tried to find a place to balance all the sorrow while still living. It took a very long time to believe I would ever find peace again. Some days were harder than others. I never knew what would trigger the emotions. As time passed, I finally allowed myself to smile again. I remember the first time I laughed. It was about two months after our son had died. I was surprised that almost immediately after laughing, I was overcome with guilt. How could I allow myself to be happy after this happened? What kind of person was I? I felt I was being disrespectful to my son.

Getting past my due date was especially challenging. I was consumed by thoughts of what should have been. The holidays, too, were difficult, but I kept trying to put my life back together. I knew that I had to, for my sanity. I went back to work. This was especially difficult because I was around laboring women and babies all day, reminding me of what I had lost. But I loved my work and couldn't imagine doing any other kind of nursing. Looking back, I think that it was this that helped me deal with all of the pain. It forced me to deal with my emotions on a daily basis and not just bury them.

Soon the good days outnumbered the bad. I remember enjoying the seasons—fall, winter, and then spring; I had missed all of them the year before when I was on bed rest. For some reason, I felt much better when spring started, like the fog had finally lifted. I felt like I had finally gotten back to "normal." But I was definitely a changed person. This experience forced me to realize the uncertainty of life. It helped me to reprioritize my life. I appreciate my family, friends, and life itself more today. I never take anything or anyone for granted. Don't get me wrong, it's not all roses. Some days are still very hard; some days I want to wallow in self-pity. And I think this is OK. I can feel sad about what happened, but I can also look beyond this and remember the good that happened. It helps me to remember the good things, like the feeling when I first found out I was pregnant, the look in my husband's eyes when I told him he was going to be a father, the first time I felt my baby move, the hopes and dreams I had for him, the love and support from my family and friends. These are the things that help me heal, and I think I am a better person and nurse today because of what I have experienced.

Healing is an ongoing process, one that I am not sure will ever end. There are many bad things that I could choose to remember, but there are also good things to remember. I feel I owe it to my son to remember him with a smile, for he brought me so much. And maybe, just maybe, that is the answer to the question *Why.*

Emotional Care of a Perinatal Loss and Its Impact on the Labor and Delivery Nurse

Brenda Whiting Beard, R.N., BSN, and Louise Ward, R.N., MSN

"Oh, you're a labor and delivery nurse? . . . That must be so much fun!" is the usual enthusiastic comment when people find out what kind of nursing I do. They might be envisioning loving Madonnas with their angelic babes all pink and healthy, with the nurse present for surrogate mothering when the moms need to rest. What a great job that would be.

The reality is that nursing at a level 3, tertiary care center is a mixture of emergency nursing, operating room nursing, an intensive care unit, some basic maternity nursing, and a large portion of teaching. My college education prepared me for that and much more. What the best education in the world cannot prepare one for is a perinatal loss—a stillborn infant or a premature delivery where all efforts fail to save the neonate's little life.

I have been enabled through education, and empowered by experience, to manage the clinical aspects of caring for a family facing a perinatal loss, but what do I do with my own sense of grief? No one ever told me that as a nurse I would grieve so deeply, and sometimes so often, with families that until recently were strangers to me. As a professional, my head knows to stay focused so I can help start the family on the right path for grieving. A complex and perhaps never-ending process at a time that should be filled with great joy. Also, as a parent, my heart tells me many other things. This is what a dear friend (and, coincidentally, my minister) calls stirring up the "pot of loss." When you are faced with a loss situation, all previous losses are stimulated. They will rise to the surface much as the ingredients rise when a soup or stew is stirred. In the process of stirring, this concoction, left so long on the back burner, is seasoned, is tasted, and a new seasoning— a new loss—is added; then it resumes simmering. A family experiencing a perinatal loss will have their "pot of loss" uncovered, and all previous losses will surface. They may remember a family member's death, the loss of a friend, the loss of a pet, or the loss of a dream. How they dealt with these events will impact on how they deal with this perinatal loss. Likewise, my "pot of loss" impacts on how I deal with them as their nurse. It is a very well seasoned pot that provides the sustenance needed to continue in a healthy way. I taste from it briefly, am strengthened, and go forward to do the work at hand.

The first thing I do when admitting a family with a loss to Labor & Delivery is to initiate a Perinatal Loss Checklist (PLC). The PLC is documentation of the events that occur and the support team involved. It is a concise list that helps the nurse stay focused while providing care. It also ensures that all team members are notified that their services may be required. The team includes the doctors (obstetrician and pediatrician), nurses, social worker, clergy, and frequently the genetics department. We work as a team, one service complementing and adding to the others' contributions. The goal is to facilitate the family's grieving. Depending on circumstances, the family may not see all members of the team while on Labor & Delivery, so the PLC also acts as a guide to the team. What is not documented at delivery will be attended to at another time prior to discharge. A copy of this form is forwarded to the attending physician's office so that the repetition of painful questions can be decreased and accurate communication of helpful information will be increased.

The PLC's most important function is to stimulate the collection of memorabilia for the family. The time spent in Labor & Delivery after birth is often the only time the family may have with the child. Whether the loss is a stillborn, a severely premature infant, or a baby born with anomalies that are incompatible with life, it is important to emphasize the act of making memories. I often make suggestions to the family that will help them plan for the delivery of their baby.

In the best of circumstances, I take the time to discuss with the family their desires for after the baby is born. They may not have any concrete plans beyond deciding whether or not to see their baby. This issue alone can be of great importance. Those who are sure they would like to see their baby make my job that much easier. I will advise the ones who are unsure to see the baby, offering to hold the infant for them while they look on, if that might make it easier for them. My most difficult task is working with a family that chooses not to see the baby at all. I respect their decision (albeit with a heavy heart that I keep to myself), and tell them that some families feel this way as a result of fear. I assure them that reality is very often less frightening than imagination. I usually take this opportunity to share some of my experiences. First of all, I state that their decision is not irrevocable, thus leaving the door open for them to change their minds. Until the mother is discharged or the baby is picked up by the designated funeral home, there is always an opportunity to see the baby in our morgue's family area. While I know that the optimal time is soon after birth, attempts are made to make the viewing as easy as possible. I also give them the benefit of my experiences with families that have contacted me to expressing regret over not having seen their babies. I feel comfortable that I am doing this in a very nonjudgmental way. When a family opts not to see their baby, I take extra time to hold this baby in private. This is one of the ways I help myself to heal after caring for a loss.

I inquire about the family's faith and their desire to meet with a member of our clergy staff. Some families have strong desires, while others may not have thought of having the baby blessed or a prayer said.

During the delivery, I try to keep the room a safe, quiet place while providing physical comfort and facilitating the birth process. I inform the physician or midwife of the wishes of the family during the labor, so that all of us are aware and sensitive to their needs.

I position myself on one side of the bed and encourage the father (or significant other) to be at the other side. If the father has expressed fear of watching the birth, I suggest that he look into his partner's eyes or toward the top of the bed. I often see fathers glancing at the delivery. I usually am ready with a blanket to take the baby from the midwife or physician and place it gently in the prepared crib. I preheat the crib and have baby blankets and towels lining it, as I would do for any infant. I cover the baby completely or partially, according to the predetermined plan. I often note that a grandparent who is in the room at this time ventures over for a closer look in the crib. Once the physical aspects of the delivery are completed—such as the delivery of the placenta and repair of the perineum—and the mother's vital signs are stable, I turn my attention to the baby.

I wipe the baby dry, taking care not to damage the skin, which may be very fragile. I do the baby care in the room of the patient as often as possible. By watching this process, the families are able to see how I handle their baby with gentle and respectful touches. I think it also helps them to see that it is acceptable to touch these babies. I am tearful at these deliveries. I cannot help but be saddened by the loss of potential life and love that this family is experiencing. I believe that my tears help to validate that this is a life worth grieving for.

I encourage the family to touch the baby as I prepare it for presentation to the mother. Sometimes I hear them comment about features that resemble those of family members. Even in babies with anomalies, there is often a trait they see as familiar. When I hand the baby to the mother, I introduce the baby as "your son" or "your daughter." I make every attempt to place this baby into the family. When the family discusses naming, I suggest that they can either use the name that they had originally chosen, or they may wish to save that name for another child and choose something different. The point is to encourage naming this baby, to help give him or her an identity within the family.

Protocol requires taking pictures of the baby both clothed and unclothed. The parents are told that this will be done and that they may take the pictures home with them. If they opt not to take the pictures home, they are kept on file with the social worker. One family returned to claim them seven years after delivery. Most likely these are the only pictures of this child, since many families do not bring cameras with them.

I try to take pictures that I would want to have. The Polaroid camera at work allows me to take multiple shots to achieve the best pictures possible within the limitations of the camera. In recent years, I have begun to photograph the actual deliveries, the blessings, and the family members with the baby. These are unposed pictures and I am careful to be as unobtrusive as possible. I also take pictures of the baby alone, using a background frame that I developed to eliminate the hospital equipment from the scene. Using stuffed animals donated by the Labor & Delivery staff, I can add a nursery atmosphere as well as use the animals to prop and pose the baby. These pictures have been very well received.

The rest of the memorabilia packet contains footprints and handprints, locks of hair, the hospital identification bands, and the blanket, T-shirt and hat that the baby wore in the pictures and while being held by the family. I also enclose a copy of *When Hello Means Goodbye* and a baby memory booklet filled in with the time and date of delivery, weight, length, and the persons involved with the patient's care.

In the future, our perinatal loss care will include, but not be limited to, follow-up phone calls at two weeks, six months, and one year, an invitation to an annual memorial service; encouraging involvement with community support groups; providing in-services training for our coworkers; and continued evaluation of and improvements to our memorabilia packet, based on input from families, coworkers, and professional journals.

The care of these special families is rewarding and extremely satisfying work. I choose to care for them as often as I can or to instruct a less experienced nurse, to allow her to grow in a nursing skill that is not always covered in a textbook. I am very fortunate to work alongside a very compassionate team who are dedicated to making this tragic road somewhat easier to travel.

A Social Worker's Perspective on Pregnancy Loss

Andrea Seigerman, MSW, LCSW

When I was asked to write about the emotional impact of pregnancy loss, I began outlining a rather lengthy, descriptive paper about phases of the grief process, stages of pregnancy, and how they interrelate. It was to have been objective and informative without being too formal or academic. As I further considered the topic and reflected on my almost twenty years of experience as a clinical social worker in an inner-city teaching hospital's obstetrics department, my focus and goal changed. I decided to write about the people—all the people—who are affected by a pregnancy loss. In this way I hope to convey the deep and far-reaching effects, impact, and impression of this kind of loss. The effects are at times unrecognized, at times invisible, and at times denied. This article is not intended to be a "how to cope" manual regarding pregnancy loss, but rather an exploration of the complex, multifaceted dynamics of pregnancy loss. It is my hope that this article will serve to inform two different groups of people—those who have and those who have not experienced a loss. By reading this article, couples who have suffered a loss will feel less alone, more connected, and better able to cope. Readers with no experience of pregnancy loss will have an understanding of the extent to which that loss affects its survivors.

What is pregnancy loss, and who are the women that experience it? For my purposes, in this paper, pregnancy loss is all-inclusive. It is early first trimester miscarriages, ectopic pregnancies, second trimester genetic terminations and natural losses, the demise of one baby in a multiple gestation, a full-term stillborn, the death of a baby soon after it is born. And who are the courageous women who suffer these losses? The group is large and diverse and spares no one. All ages, religions, races, income levels, and stages of life are represented. Imagine these women, united in loss but as different from each other as one could expect: twelve-year-olds who aren't even clear about how they got pregnant, "older" women who are pregnant for the first time, single or married or divorced women, women with unplanned or unwanted pregnancies, women who have been trying to conceive for years. Each and every one of them, utilizing her own life experience, support network, and understanding of the medical problems, will have to cope and move on.

How does one understand the impact of a loss? In part, by assessing the value of what has been lost. The word "pregnancy" conjures up images of smiling, gurgling babies, tired, bleary-eyed adults, and a "glowing pregnant woman." It is a word that epitomizes joy, hope for the future, dreams and relationships yet to be realized, and perhaps the next step on the ladder of life—parenthood. For some people, it represents the fulfillment of a lifelong goal. Expectant fathers share and experience this early emotional connection along with their partners. They often take great pride in considering their soon-to-be role, their contribution to society, and the mark their child will leave on the world. In Rodgers and Hammerstein's *Carousel,* the leading man sings "My Boy Bill," a song anticipating, savoring, and worrying about his upcoming new role and responsibilities. Many health care professionals who choose to work in this specialty area do so because it is considered a "happy" job. For everyone involved in "pregnancy," there seems to be an abundance of positive energy invested in it, committed to it, expected of it. Pregnancy, from a nonmedical, societal perspective, is considered a simple and natural part of life. Getting pregnant, staying pregnant, and then delivering a healthy, bouncing baby is the way it's supposed to be.

Undoubtedly, then, we can understand the utter devastation felt by people when there is a pregnancy loss. Parents feel cheated out of a wondrous, natural experience that was to be theirs. Suddenly their dreams are shattered and their hope for a family is lost or temporarily put on hold. Instead of going to baby showers and decorating rooms, they are planning funerals and putting baby items away. This is not what's supposed to happen. Your baby isn't supposed to pass on before you have had a chance to hold, love, care for it, and share in its life. Mothers and fathers alike express shock, numbness, sadness, emptiness, anger (at G-d, at life, at others who have healthy children), and confusion: "I keep thinking this is just a bad dream, and when I wake up, I'll still be pregnant." They just don't understand why something so natural, pure, and simple has slipped out of their grasp. Bereaved parents sometimes allude to a loss of focus and direction, an inability to know what to do next. "I got the room ready and quit my job so I could be home with my baby. I was planning to spend my time raising my child. What do I do now?"

Feelings of guilt, blame, and failure may also begin to surface. While these last few reactions have no basis in reality, mothers often feel ultimately responsible for the well-being of their unborn child, and therefore culpable. They review events leading up to the loss, seeking an answer, a cause, a reason. Sometimes they unfortunately settle on an action or lack of action of their own as the causative factor. Women often think, If only I hadn't carried those heavy grocery bags. If only I had rested more. If I had eaten better and gotten more exercise. If I hadn't been so nervous and worried so much. All these ruminations lead to the same conclusion: I didn't take good enough care of my baby. Feelings of failure can arise out of comparisons: None of my friends had any problems with their pregnancies. We went to the same doctor and exercise classes. She works, too, and probably doesn't sleep any more than I do. All of which leads to, What's the matter with me? How come I can't do this simple thing? It is not uncommon for their partners to go through a similar process. Many men have shared these comments with me: If I'd helped more around the house, she could have rested. Maybe we should have waited longer. Maybe I shouldn't have pushed for a baby so soon.

The context in which the loss is perceived by the mother and her ability to freely communicate how she is feeling may contribute to her long-term adjustment. A not uncommon, although rarely discussed, response to the ending of a pregnancy is a sense of relief. Women don't readily share such "unacceptable" thoughts as This just wasn't the right time for me to have a baby, but I never considered abortion or adoption as an alternative. For some women, now that a baby won't be coming, life can continue on its originally intended course—a continuation of school, beginning a new job, getting out of a bad relationship, struggling to balance existing parental and child care stresses. Relief may coexist equally with feelings of sadness and grief. For some women the situation is even more complex: I used to think about how much easier it would be if I weren't pregnant, if somehow it would just disappear and things could go back to normal. Now my wish has come true, and I feel like I killed my baby. It's vitally important for parents to have the opportunity to talk, without hesitation, to their partners and to supportive family members, friends, and health care providers about their conflicting feelings regarding the loss of their baby.

Parents are not alone at the time of a pregnancy loss. The members of the team who are caring for the patient often experience a similar flood of reactions and emotions. After all, isn't it their job and commitment to guide a woman safely from the beginning to the end of a pregnancy, to check and recheck to make sure there aren't any problems, to anticipate problems that might occur, and to resolve medical complications that do arise? However, sometimes even all their caring, attention and use of modern technology can't stave off the inevitable. We can certainly comprehend why they may not want to be the ones to confirm a bad diagnosis, a poor prognosis, or the absence of a fetal heartbeat. But it must be done. They have to communicate the news, answer the questions if possible, and watch the looks of shock and despair come over the faces of their patients. It would be foolhardy to think that this does not take a toll. Caregivers may (and do) cry along with the parents, feel upset, feel responsible, wish they could take away the hurt, review their work to see if there's anything they could have missed, wonder how much longer they can do this kind of work, talk with colleagues for support, or busy themselves with work and move on—pushing away the feelings. After all, they're only human. For everyone involved— patient, partner, care provider—there may be a sense that the situation is out of their control, that in spite of everyone's best effort this pregnancy, this life, was lost.

As time goes on, bereaved parents may be viewed as being at the center of the crisis of pregnancy loss and its impact on daily life. Just as a pebble dropped into water generates concentric circles, the effect and impact of pregnancy loss spreads out to touch many people in more ways and for longer periods of time than one might imagine. Having already discussed the reactions of the mother and father, I want to look at the first circle. The parents, children, other family members, and close friends of the bereaved come to mind. These are the people who would have been the grandparents, siblings, aunts, uncles, cousins, pals of the baby. They have already shared with the parents in the growth and development of the unborn child, have seen the ultrasound pictures, and have felt the baby move and kick. Some may have offered to loan cribs and baby clothes, offered to baby-sit, begun to knit a blanket or sweater, or offered to share their toys and even their room. Now they have to shift gears and direct their efforts to providing comfort, support, a listening ear, a calming touch—to helping in whatever way they can. While the expectant mother or couple eagerly accepted previous offers of services and goods, how will they now respond to offers of emotional support and to being taken care of? Over the years I have found that people strive to be independent, capable, and self-sufficient, and want to be so considered by others, especially in times of crisis. Will the bereaved parents accept help from those who want to give it?

What about the children who would have been siblings or cousins? What do you say? How do you explain the passing of a baby to a youngster eagerly awaiting its arrival? If there is a funeral, should the older children attend? Is there a way to be clear and truthful about the loss without making it sound too frightening? Although they are in the midst of their own grief, parents are concerned about the other children at home, who want to know that Mommy is OK and when the baby is coming home. Parents have to continue as caregivers while requiring care themselves. Parents generally want to discuss these questions and are open to suggestions. Often the family pediatrician can be very helpful in framing answers to the questions children inevitably ask.

Continuing the flow out from the center, you next encounter neighbors, coworkers, classmates, the people from your congregation, local shop keepers, and so on. A whole new set of concerns arises. How many of them knew about the pregnancy, are pregnant themselves, or have young infants? How does one explain what happened to concerned and curious associates? How much should you say and how much do they really want to know? How will you face it when their due date arrives? Should you go to the baby shower you've been invited to next week? Your daily acquaintances are undoubtedly as unsure as you are. They don't want to upset, ignore, or anger parents by anything they might say or do. These are delicate situations, and we all have to act or respond as best we can. There are no simple answers.

On the outer perimeter and on a more global scale, pregnancy and babies are everywhere. So, just when bereaved parents feel composed and ready to face the world, they are bombarded by TV commercials for Pampers, pregnant women in the supermarket, and babies in the park. One can't escape the realities of birth and death, pregnancy and its loss. Each day women, their partners, and their families move ahead and (hopefully) grow stronger as they recover from the complexities of pregnancy loss. Many may connect with local support groups. Support groups and books on pregnancy loss are excellent ways to increase one's understanding of the topic and to receive ongoing encouragement, motivation, and strength. A few clinical snapshots will dramatically illustrate the depth and breadth of the impact of pregnancy loss.

A young Hispanic couple wants a photo of their anomalous stillborn to send to their parents in Puerto Rico so the family can better understand what happened. A thirty-year-old woman and her husband softly discuss what to tell Molly, their three-year-old daughter, who is waiting at home with a teddy bear for her baby brother. An Asian man with a stoic, expressionless face sits beside his silent wife, whose face is streaked with tears. A sixteen-year-old boy approaches his parents, wanting to ask about the family secret—his twin brother who died at birth. A fifty-year-old only child with ailing, aging parents wonders what things might be like if her mother's two fetal losses hadn't occurred and she was now the oldest of three. A labor and delivery nurse who has just learned she is pregnant is assigned to care for a woman with a fetal demise. A twenty-five-year-old woman, mother of a five-year-old, suffers a second trimester loss and becomes suicidal because she feels she's let everyone down.

In closing, it would be difficult and unfair to define, catalog, or quantify the emotional impact of pregnancy loss in any standardized way. The reactions to loss are as unique and special as are the people involved. Loss touches people in many different ways, and at times for years into the future. There is a fluid process of adjustment, reflection, and acceptance—at times easier, at times more difficult. The child is gone but never forgotten, and often is the subject of continued fantasies about what might have been.

Perspectives of a Newborn Special Care Unit Nurse

Laurel Jonason, R.N., BSN

What is it like in a Newborn Special Care Unit? It is many things. Some of our activities have been featured on TV shows that talk about ethical issues, expensive medical care, and sometimes the medical miracles which often happen there. For those of us who work in these units, our job is multifaceted, too. It can be incredibly intense as the staff struggles, with all of our combined expertise, to save a small life. It can be rewarding when we can watch a baby who was deathly ill finally go home to his or her family. It can also be agonizingly sad when, in spite of all our efforts, a baby dies.

All the babies who come to our unit are alive. Those children who are stillborn or are delivered before an age for which any resuscitation can be done are cared for by the Labor & Delivery staff. Often, since we are a tertiary center, we receive babies from other hospitals, sent to us for the type of specialized care that only a few hospitals can provide. The babies we receive can be premature, have physical defects or heart problems, have experienced a very difficult delivery, or have a need for specialized ventilation therapy that is not available at other hospitals.

So what is my job in all of this? The easiest way to describe it is to relate the events in the life of one of the many babies I have cared for. This is an actual case that I have disguised to protect the privacy of the family involved. Tom was a full-term baby. He was the firstborn child of a married couple, Luis and Carmen. He was born at an outlying hospital and transported to us for worsening respiratory distress. When I received him and became Tom's primary nurse, I could see that we would have to fight very hard for this child. Tom was diagnosed as having persistent pulmonary hypertension, a situation in which the baby's lungs remain in their fetal state and do not allow for proper oxygenation of the blood. He had a tube in his windpipe, and we began to turn up the settings of his ventilator. Meanwhile, Tom was in shock and I rapidly prepared and administered the many syringes of fluid and medication to try and support his blood pressure. The attending physicians and the house staff made the decision to approach the family for consent to use nitric oxide, which has allowed many babies with this condition to "open up" their lungs and be ventilated. They spoke to the parents, and after explaining Tom's condition and the treatment they wanted to try, the parents agreed. As we began the nitric oxide and continued the high-frequency ventilation, Tom was deteriorating. As I drew and sent each new blood gas, we all hoped for an improvement. Preliminary lab results told us that Tom probably had a blood infection. He had already been started on antibiotics, and as I prepared his second dose, I hoped that this round would help us turn the corner. The doctors ordered, and I mixed, new drugs to help Tom's heart push against the resistance of his stiff lungs. More fluid was pushed. Blood products were given. The doctors talked about Extra Corporeal Membrane Oxygenation (ECMO), a type of bypass pump that could act as part of Tom's lungs until they could get better. We needed time—time to get an ECMO team together, time to get the parents in to see their baby, time to allow the antibiotics to work, time to call in social services, time. . . . And it was running out . . . and then we knew . . . what we had feared all along . . . that we would not save this child. . . . Perhaps this is the most difficult time for us as staff members . . . to know that we tried so hard, and no matter what we did, it was not enough. Some people would now say, "There is nothing more we can do," but there is . . . and in that moment, which sometimes comes collectively and sometimes separately, we all had to redefine our goals. We needed to try to keep Tom alive until his parents arrived. We needed a little time to prepare the parents as best we could for the death of their child. We needed to find the best way to support a couple who had just had a birth and would now have a death.

Luis and Carmen arrived in time. As gently as they could, team explained that we had done all we could, but Tom was dying. His heart rate was dropping, and he would die soon. We asked them if they wanted Tom baptized, and all the staff gathered at Tom's bedside as the priest baptized him and prayed for support for the parents. The attending physician and I remained at Tom's bedside. Together we explained what choices there were for Tom's final minutes. This is always a difficult thing to do. We ask parents to choose from options that none of us what. Do they want their baby to die in his bed on all the life support? Do they want to hold him while he is still on all the equipment? Do they want to remove him from the life support and hold him as he dies? Do they want to hold him in the ICU or go to a private room? What we try to do is to offer them a "road map" for a territory where they have never been. They can choose which direction to go . . . we will be there to help and support. Luis and Carmen asked about what would happen when Tom died. We explained that we would give him a small amount of morphine to make him comfortable . . . that his heart would slow even more . . . that he might breathe a few times on his own . . . and then he would be still . . . and, they could hold him as long as they wanted. We asked if there was anyone else they wanted called. They said that Carmen's parents were on the way. We alerted the secretary to let us know as soon as they arrived. Luis and Carmen wanted a chance to hold Tom before he died. Since we believed that he would die quickly off life support, we curtained off Tom's section of the nursery and moved all of his equipment to allow his parents to hold him. Luis and Carmen wept as their new son was placed in their arms for the first time. As the monitors showed

Tom's vital signs continuing to dwindle, his parents told us it was time to remove those last connections, which seemed to be merely prolonging their child's dying. We escorted Luis and Carmen into a private room near the nursery, and all of Tom's caregivers worked together to remove the life support. Tom, free of all his tubes and wires, was gently wrapped in a warm blanket and dressed in a clean shirt and hat, than taken to his parents. Tom was still alive as I placed him in his parents' arms. At the parents' request, the priest returned and Tom's grandparents arrived in time to hear the priest's blessing. As the parents murmured to Tom, he took a single gasp and was still. Luis asked if Tom was "gone"; the attending physician listened and said "Yes."

We have a protocol in our unit for what to do when a baby dies. It serves as a guideline for our actions, but much of what happens next is determined by the wishes and needs of the family. We offer them our presence but also give them the option of being alone. We allow supporting friends and family to be present if the parents wish. We encourage the parents to see and hold their child, but we respect their right to refuse—some parents find holding their baby at the time of death is just too difficult. We explain to the parents that the staff can hold their baby instead—and if this is what the parents wish, we will hold the child until death has occurred. We often offer the parents the option of bathing and dressing their baby—if they choose not to, their baby is always bathed and dressed before it leaves our unit. We prepare a "bereavement packet" that has a memory book for footprints and handprints, locks of hair, and mementos. We include several pictures of the baby—the setting and style of the photos are the choice of the parents. Often we take pictures of the parents holding the baby as well as close-ups of their child. The bereavement packet also contains literature about grief, lists of support groups, a bibliography, and additional materials.

Luis and Carmen held Tom for over an hour. Carmen's parents held him, too, and then left Luis and Carmen alone with Tom. They had expressed the wish to be alone for a while, so we agreed that I would come back when they called me. After this period, I returned to them and explained the contents of the bereavement packet. Our social worker had spent some time with them and had discussed burial options. Although some parents refuse the packet (we keep it on file in case they want it later), Carmen and Luis wanted their packet. They wanted to see Tom after I bathed and redressed him, so I tenderly washed Tom and put him in clean clothes. I also obtained Tom's handprints and footprints as well as a lock of his hair, and I placed these inside the memory book, along with his crib card and name sign. After I brought Tom back to his parents, they held him for a few minutes more and said their last good-byes. They had discussed their wishes regarding autopsy with the attending physician and had signed the necessary paperwork. Luis and Carmen handed Tom back to me—this is always a hard moment for all of us. I hugged them both . . . and then they left their precious child with me and walked out of the unit. I prepared Tom for his final journey, and then he was gone from my care. I returned to his empty bed. I paused to reflect on his short life and to review all the events that had occurred. As always, I hoped that I had done my best to meet the needs of his family. My efforts to support this family had a cost for me. A death is draining—I would need to "refill my cup." I have experienced so many deaths in our unit, and I know how important this personal restoration is— each if us has to replenish our "compassion stores" before we can best care for the next family who needs us. Sometimes this is hard to do.

As bereavement chairperson for our unit, I do much of the nursing follow-up on families who have had a baby die in our unit. As I do for all the families, I prepared and sent a sympathy card to Luis and Carmen. I added them to the list that we keep, and the following March I sent them an invitation to our Night of Remembrance, to which we invite all the families of children who have died at the hospital in the last two years. It sometimes overwhelms me as I send out the invitations. Each name is a personal loss to that family . . . and there are so many that I was there for. Luis and Carmen came to our remembrance ceremony. As Tom's name was read, I handed a flower to Carmen, who had come forward to receive it. At the reception afterward, I talked to both of these parents with whom I had shared a short but intense and meaningful experience. They were going to a support group and said that they had good and bad days. The holidays were tough . . . but they had hope that maybe next year, when they were invited again, Carmen might be pregnant. I told them to call me if they needed me. I shared with them the short life of their child . . . I would remember him, too.

Family Grief and Recovery Process When a Baby Dies

Leena Väisänen, MD, PhD

The loss of a baby is always traumatic. The crisis begins with traumatic experiences. The parents transit into the liminal space between life and death. This stage also underlines the paradoxical quality of grief. A logical thought is followed by another, which contradicts the first. For instance, the mother feels she cannot respond at all, because she feels dead herself. She cannot be alive, because her baby is dead. Recovery also seems something impossible and far away, although ideas of recovery appear early on in the process, balancing the mind and necessarily protecting the ego from being split. The subliminal time of grief is shown in the altered way of experiencing things. One lives in an altered time with strange symbols, omens, and dreams, and unusual psychic and physical experiences. The experience of grief is not only stepwise and processual, but multivoiced and stratified, like counterpoint in music, and there is reciprocal movement within it like paradoxical loops. The loss of a baby results in grief that runs counter to the expectations. The parents have invested so much primeval energy in the baby who is no longer alive that they tend to re-create her/him in their minds psychologically or spiritually. Grieving thus involves deep attachment rather than detachment, and the processing of this attachment makes it possible to recover.

THE SOMATIC ASPECT OF GRIEF

Family grief requires collective tolerance and sharing. The family members huddle close together and set up a wailing wall around them: it is permissible at home to cry aloud or grieve quietly. The quiet, largely somatic aspect of grief is strongly present after baby loss. The mother, and occasionally also the father, may find themselves in a subliminal space between life and death, where the pain of the loss, emptiness, and longing is present as physical pain. The loss of a baby in the symbiotic phase results in grief manifested as physical pain and longing, feelings of emptiness, strange sensations, and a phantom baby. Some mothers are able to verbalize this better, but all losses involve feelings of distress, restlessness, pain, and anxiety which are due to the fact that the mother, with all her finely tuned physiological systems, was intended to keep her baby alive. Although there is no baby, the mother's psychophysiological need to care tends to persist. She is still symbiotically dependent on her baby, who no longer exists as a living being.

She is constantly preoccupied with the baby, the grave, and death. She may even be so intensely dependent on the grave that she cannot leave the locality. Visiting the grave daily may be important, and even when she does not actually visit the grave, she may be conscious of it. Because the baby is in a grave, the mother may feel for a long time that she is in a grave herself. Phantom babies are symbolic representations of grief and continue their nearly physical existence in the family. The alternative religious metaphor is a baby angel, which splits the traumatic experience in two: the disconcerting body of the baby in the grave and a consoling angel. Grief reflects the psychological and spiritual attachment to the baby that was lost physically and strongly resists abandonment of the baby. It is based on the primeval energy of parental attachment, which is used, although there is no baby.

GRIEF OF FAMILY MEMBERS

The mother's grief process and recovery are reflected in the family's overall coping. If the mother is able to share her attachment to the future baby early in the pregnancy, the father is able to support his wife after their bereavement. Fathers are generally the best supporters for their wives. The challenge posed by grief to the father is a need to find his own specific grief beyond the mother's grief. In the light of the present findings, young parents who lose their first child need a lot of support. They may have an inadequate support network, having moved to a new locality as students, for example. They have abundant experiences of being left alone. The families who already had a strong social network were given adequate outside support of many kinds. It is important in these families to be able to be alone from time to time. Children were the active parties who interpreted and commented on their parents, and who used their energy and imagination to console their parents by all possible means. A child may also assume the role of a therapist in relation to her/his parents. In this study group, latency age girls who had identified with their mother's pregnancy appeared to be at risk, because they also symbolically lost the baby or identified with the baby and began to fear for their own death. Children may also have transient age-appropriate symptoms and therefore need an adult to talk about things that are important for them. The basic attitude of children toward death and dead people is natural and curious. Children are conscious of the paradoxical quality of their parents' grief, because they share a cyclic notion of time and way of reasoning. Children are also able to delay their own grief reaction to help their parents.

TIME OF GRIEF

Grieving takes a lot of time. Although the restlessness, anxiety, and depressive moods disappear, grief continues as a long process. The first year is the worst. Each parent has her/his individual schedule. Grief is not something that becomes linearly alleviated, but rather is a circular process that is activated by the intense initial guilt and obsessive need to find out causes and details. This study showed the recovery times to vary, depending on the individual personalities of the parents and the family structure. The family recovery process mostly takes place through dialogue between the family members, which allows them to find new meanings. Their goal is to survive the catastrophe by finding new meanings for the family security system, their identity as a family, and their worldview. The very short recovery times reported in quantitative studies reflect their short follow-up times and the research setup. In this study the active grief time lasted usually for two or three years. Grief for the death of a baby continues at some level forever, although it is not pathological or complicated. When time elapses, the feelings of pain are alleviated.

Perspectives of a Genetic Counselor

Leslie Ciarlegio, MS

The prospect of meeting with a genetic counselor can be intimidating for the client. There are often fears associated with the investigation of one's own makeup in the most basic sense. People also often have misconceptions of what genetic counseling is all about. As technological knowledge expands, and the genetic basis for common disorders is understood, it becomes increasingly likely that the "average" person will have the occasion to speak with a genetic counselor. Ideally, this sneak peek into genetic counseling will help to alleviate the anxiety of the unknown and help clients to prepare for a more productive genetic counseling session.

WHAT IS GENETIC COUNSELING?

The American Society of Human Genetics (ASHG) defines genetic counseling in the following way:

Genetic counseling is a communication process which deals with the human problems associated with the occurrence, or the risk of occurrence, of a genetic disorder in a family. This process involves an attempt by one or more appropriately trained persons to help the individual or family

1. comprehend the medical facts, including the diagnosis, the probable course of the disorder, and the available management;
2. appreciate the way heredity contributes to the disorder, and the risk of recurrence;
3. understand the options for dealing with the risk of recurrence;
4. choose the course of action which seems appropriate to them in view of their risk and their family goals, and act in accordance with that decision; and
5. make the best possible adjustment to the disorder in an affected family member and/or the risk of recurrence of that disorder.

WHO ARE GENETIC COUNSELORS?

Genetic counselors are members of a health care team. They provide information and support to families and serve as patient advocates. They are also educators and a resource for other health professionals and for the public. Genetic counseling has historically been provided by physicians, social workers, and nurses. Currently, the majority of genetic counselors are professionals who have prepared through accredited programs focusing on the combination of medical genetics and psychology. Counselors are certified through the American Board of Genetic Counseling, which was established in 1993. Previously, certification was through the American Board of Medical Genetics.

Genetic counselors have become highly subspecialized: there are counselors who specialize in prenatal genetics, pediatric genetics, or adult genetics. Some counselors work in commercial labs as liaisons with the referring community. Some counselors work in research settings. Some counselors work only with patients affected with specific disease types, such as inborn errors of metabolism, neuro-genetics, or cancer genetics. Others work in a single disease clinic, such as a cystic fibrosis center. Private practice is also a growing area for genetic counselors. As the Human Genome Project further uncovers the genetic basis for many "common" diseases, genetic counselors will be found more globally in medical practice.

GENERAL PRINCIPLES OF GENETIC COUNSELING

In the ASHG definition, genetic counseling is described as a communication process. This implies participation of both counselor and client. Such a strategy is often unfamiliar to many patients, and this unfamiliarity can create anxiety for them. This may also be a new approach for many physicians. In this new role, the patient assumes responsibility for his or her actions. In order for the counselor/client relationship to be effective, and to encourage patient participation, the style and dialogue in a genetic counseling session must be tailored to each client's needs, goals, and perspective. Nondirectiveness is a fundamental principle of genetic counseling. This refers to the belief that clients are capable, if thoroughly informed, of making appropriate choices for themselves. Counselors need not, and should not, make decisions for their patients. Nondirectiveness is essential. Ethnicity and socioeconomic background have to be considered. Ideally, a genetic counselor will maintain "unconditional positive regard" toward the patient, as well as continuous sensitivity to the patient's varying emotional states. Without these considerations, the counselor cannot elicit all relevant information and will not be able to transmit information effectively.

It has been said that genetic counseling is 20% genetics and 80% counseling, and I would agree. The purpose of genetic counseling is education of patients, but also their empowerment, advocacy, and support.

Genetic counseling is often crisis intervention. Patients may be asked to deal with or to make decisions with significant and perhaps lifelong implications in a time of emotional upheaval. Issues surrounding medical interventions in pregnancy certainly fall into this category. Deciding whether or not to undergo a particular prenatal test can be very stressful. This pales in comparison, however, to deciding about what to do when faced with abnormal diagnostic test results. Many health care providers have worked with couples in these situations. However, few can truly understand their feelings and their pain. Genetic counselors are trained to appreciate the psychological aspects of these patient dilemmas.

THE GENETIC COUNSELING SESSION

Who Are Genetic Counseling Patients?

In this context of prenatal diagnosis and testing, I would like to outline a "typical" genetic counseling session. To touch briefly on an enormous subject, prenatal genetic testing has become an issue that, at some time, almost all pregnant patients face. Testing is available in many forms, at different times in gestation. First trimester genetic diagnosis is a relatively new area in obstetrics and represents the cutting edge of prenatal testing. Ultrasound at approximately ten weeks' gestation (counting from the first day of the last menstrual period) can confirm viability and the number of gestational sacs, and identify certain major structural anomalies, such as fetal anencephaly, in skilled hands. Also, screening for chromosomal abnormalities by looking at the nuchal area at this early gestational age is becoming more widely used. Second trimester genetic testing is more familiar to most patients. This includes maternal blood tests such as the AFP test or the "triple" screen, which is used to determine whether a patient appears to have a relatively high or low risk for certain chromosomal abnormalities or other birth defects. Level II ultrasound, also known as targeted fetal ultrasound, provides a detailed look at the fetal anatomy. With advancements in technology, ultrasound has become an increasingly relied upon tool in pregnancy management. Referrals for fetal echocardiography, a subspecialty of fetal ultrasound, have also increased. Amniocentesis is an invasive diagnostic procedure that can provide information about the fetal chromosome pattern. Additionally, specific hereditary conditions can be tested for through biochemical or DNA analysis.

All of these tests allow for identification of congenital anomalies or syndromes in a previable fetus. In the prenatal setting, parents may seek genetic counseling in consideration of some of this testing in an apparently normal pregnancy. Less commonly, parents may meet with a genetic counselor to help them at a time when this testing has identified a problem in a pregnancy.

Content of a Genetic Counseling Session

For pregnancy-related issues, as outlined above, there are in general two types of genetic counseling sessions: those where parents are concerned about potential risks and outcomes, and those where patients are concerned about a known problem with the pregnancy. Despite the vastly different natures of these sessions, there are common aspects. Any counseling session has two major components: the provision of information to the client, and a therapeutic dialogue where the counselor listens to, hears, and responds to the patient's reactions to this information.

The Structure of a Session

Most genetic counseling sessions are scheduled by telephone and conducted in person. It is occasionally necessary to have these discussions over the telephone, but this is not optimal. Ideally, there is a private room specifically designated for counseling purposes with adequate seating for the genetic counselor, the client(s), and any other people the client feels are appropriate to have there. In a medical center, the genetic counselor may include students or other health care providers who are interested in observing a genetic counseling session. Of course, this should be done only with the patient's permission. Patients have every right to decline the presence of observers, especially in what can be a very emotionally charged session.

Initially, the genetic counselor will go through the process of "contracting" with the patient. This refers to outlining the session to establish common objectives. Patients may be asked how much they know and understand already. Especially in the situation of a known fetal anomaly, patients come to genetic counseling with wide variation in the amount of information they have been given before this session. Patients are often asked what their expectations are and what they hope to achieve in the session. The counselor will provide the patient with a general overview of the session that should take these expectations into account. By establishing common objectives and finding out what the patient knows and wants to know, the counselor helps to ensure that the client's needs are met and the session is productive for all involved.

Most genetic counseling sessions include gathering family history information from the client. This may be as simple as a few general questions about the patient's health, family tree, and ethnic background. As the situation dictates, however, obtaining family history information may be much more involved, such as constructing a pedigree (a medical family tree) with detailed medical information about extended family members. Family history information is important in assessing potential risks in healthy patients, as well as for increasing our understanding of a known problem in a pregnancy. Knowing in advance that this information will be discussed, the patient can prepare for the genetic counseling session by gathering relevant family history information. In a prenatal setting, the genetic counselor will also inquire about potential exposures to the pregnancy, including maternal illness, prescription and over-the-counter medications, recreational drugs, and environmental exposures.

Next, most discussions will focus on the issues at hand—concerns about risks or counseling about a specific diagnosis. Throughout this part of the discussion, the counselor will often ask the patient if the information is being presented clearly. Important points will often be repeated and written down. If this is not done, ask that it be done. Many counselors draw diagrams to help illustrate their points. Pamphlets and other patient literature are commonly provided. A genetic counselor recognizes that it is difficult for families to retain all of the detailed medical information at a time of emotional upheaval. Written materials for the patient to take home can serve as a useful review, as does a follow-up phone call. In some situations, the counselor will provide the patients with a summary letter of their session as a reference for them.

Recognizing and responding to a patient's feelings are an integral part of the genetic counseling session. All clients present to genetic counseling with some level of anxiety, even in the most routine of circumstances. This seems to be particularly true in the prenatal setting. The risk for a problem, or the diagnosis of a specific anomaly in a pregnancy, is often the realization of any parent's biggest fear—"something wrong with the baby." This anxiety can be overwhelming and often has a significant impact on a patient's self-image. Additionally, it is appropriate to include in a genetic counseling session a discussion of "what ifs" regarding different potential outcomes. This allows clients to consider how they might feel in different situations, and to assess their own coping strategies and support mechanisms should a problem be identified.

Last, a plan is agreed upon. The goal of any genetic counseling session is to allow the patients to achieve a good enough understanding of their situation to make their own informed decisions. In general, there are no right or wrong answers; patients choose a course of action that is most appropriate for them and for their family goals. Counselors are often asked "What would you do?" in a variety of situations. It is unfair to the patient to answer that question directly, because there is such great variation in every individual's perspective, needs, and goals. The genetic counselor may instead review issues that would help the patients come to their own decision. The genetic counselor will act as a facilitator, but should not make decisions for patients.

To follow up, as mentioned above, the genetic counselor often telephones a client a few days after a session. At times, patients call the counselor with questions they "forgot to ask" or for clarification of certain points. Patients should be encouraged to write down their questions and concerns. It is especially difficult for clients to remember everything they want to ask in what is often an emotionally charged environment.

SUMMARY

In summary, genetic counselors provide a wide range of services as members of a health care team. The goal of genetic counseling is to provide patient education, support, advocacy, and continuity. As the availability and range of genetic testing increase, genetic counselors are found in ever expanding roles. Additionally, more and more people will be offered the option of meeting with a genetic counselor. I hope that this option may be looked upon as an opportunity . . . an opportunity for patients to gain an understanding of their own genetic issues and concerns, which will empower them to become active participants in their own health care.

A Thought from a Newborn Special Care Unit Nurse

Julia Bishop-Hahlo, R.N.

This poem was written in memory of a very special little boy, Lamar. I was his primary nurse and cared for him during the two and a half months that he was with us. He was born at 26 weeks to a drug-addicted mom. She visited him once or twice and was not involved in his care. Because she chose to remain at a distance, I allowed myself to become very attached to Lamar and he became very special to me. He, in turn, was comforted by my voice and my touch. I held him as he died, and he continues to hold a special place in my heart.

Startled and fascinated by the beauty and fragility
of your wings, I watch as you move
so gently,
so quietly,
almost unexpectedly,
through my world.
And then I watch as you move on,
fluttering softly into the distance.
Pleading silently, I beg you,
Please . . . don't go.
I haven't yet had the time
to memorize,
to remember,
to understand
the uniqueness of the beauty that is yours.
I know I cannot hold you for long,
capturing you for my world.
But, rest gently with me,
if only for a moment,
that I may treasure the memory
and the beauty of the gift that you are.

A Physician Writes of Birth and Loss

Frank H. Boehm, MD

Like most professions, medicine has its boring and mundane times. But several years ago, as I sat overlooking Niagara Falls, I reflected back on the times when being a physician was exciting and rewarding with moments filled with awe and wonder.

Eleven years ago, I was called to a hospital's labor and delivery suite to take care of a patient carrying quintuplets. Although only 24 weeks pregnant, my patient was in premature labor. Despite vigorous attempts to stop her progress, she was about to bring into this world, not one but five new human beings.

Moving her quickly into the delivery room, I knew we were in trouble because these five babies were four months premature and had only a one-in-five chance of survival. If they survived, each child would need intensive and expert care for an extended period of time in our newborn nursery.

Within minutes, I was standing in my place, ready to deliver the first quintuplet. Gazing around the room, I noticed the enormous amount of equipment and personnel. Each of the five newborn resuscitation tables brought to our arena of life and death had three newborn personnel waiting for their turn to receive one of the quintuplets. A certain amount of apprehension could easily be seen on their faces.

At the head of the patient's table were three anesthesia personnel prepared to do what was needed to bring this new litter of children into the world. Circulating around our place of birth were two obstetric nurses readying the room for our big event, and standing with me were three obstetric resident physicians.

One resident was constantly monitoring the small and fragile babies within the uterus with an ultrasound machine, while the other two stood fully scrubbed, ready to aid me. Standing in the corner were two medical students, eyes wide open in absolute amazement at what they were about to witness. Finally, sitting quietly next to his wife was the father-to-be, staring with disbelief at the spectacle he had helped to create. Despite all of these people, the room was relatively quiet. It was a quiet I had heard before—a quiet that said, "This is it—this is what our job is all about!" One at a time, they began their journey down the birth canal. Head first, Stephen appeared, followed by his siblings—Stephanie, Clinton, Barbara, and Christopher—each taking its turn to follow the previous one. As each child fell into my waiting arms, I carefully cut the umbilical cord and handed the child to a waiting pediatric team member. Finally, it was over. What seemed like an hour was in reality only a few minutes. I had just delivered five tiny human beings into this world. I was truly filled with awe and wonder.

While every birth can easily be described as awe-inspiring, after delivering more than 4,000 babies in my lifetime, there can be a certain amount of routine. But not this time. While I delivered many twins and perhaps a dozen triplets in my career, I had never delivered any quintuplets. Since spontaneous occurrence of quintuplets is approximately one in 15 million pregnancies, it is an extraordinarily rare and unique event. After the deliveries, awe and wonder filed the room. We were all a part of nature's wonder. What a privilege and honor for us all. But the human uterus is made for only one child at a time, and multiple births cause problems for both mother and babies. In this case, our excitement was soon followed by disappointment and sorrow as we helplessly watched Stephanie, Clinton, Barbara, and Christopher lose their fight for life.

What I felt that night years ago went beyond mere awe and wonder. It included humility. Being a part of such an incredible event of nature can easily bring forth such a feeling. How small and insignificant we humans are in comparison to nature's wonder. When I last saw the one surviving child, Stephen, a healthy, happy, and loving child, the feeling of humility quickly returned. It is the same humble feeling I felt while viewing up close the magnificent Niagara Falls in all its incredible splendor.

PART III
REASONS FOR THE MOST COMMON PERINATAL LOSSES

Pregnancy Loss in the First Trimester

Michael R. Berman, MD

As extraordinary as it might sound, at least 15% of clinically recognizable pregnancies end in fetal loss. Ten percent of women with no history will incur a loss, 16% after having 1 loss, 25% after 2 losses, and 45% after 3 losses. Forty percent of couples with recurrent loss have no demonstrable etiology.

We can separate losses into several different categories but for clarity I will classify them temporally throughout the pregnancy as

1. First trimester—conception through 13 weeks;

2. Second trimester—14 weeks through 26 weeks;

3. Third trimester—27 weeks through 40 weeks (term).

The most frequent losses occur in the first trimester as either spontaneous abortions (miscarriages) or ectopic pregnancies. Fifty to sixty percent of all tissue from miscarriages demonstrates chromosomal abnormalities. Five percent of these are from translocations that may be repetitive. Other common chromosome rearrangements that cause losses are Trisomies, Turner's Syndrome, triploidy (e.g., 69, XXY—17% of chromosomal abnormalities) and Tetraploidy.

These aberrations occur early in embryonic development and many times do not even manifest a fetus. Unless one or both parents are carrying an abnormal chromosome, the risk of recurrence for these early miscarriages is low. Implantation (the establishment of a maternal/fetal unit) can be interrupted by a deficiency or imbalance in the production of maternal hormones, most often progesterone from the ovary and thyroxin from the thyroid gland. Maternal bacterial, viral or viral-like infections have also been associated with first trimester pregnancy losses up to 18% of the time. In particular are mycoplasma, ureaplasma, chlamydia, and gonorrhea.

Mycoplasma can cause recurrent spontaneous abortions, whereas chlamydia and gonorrhea can also infect the uterus and fallopian tubes and damage the very delicate lining of the tubes (tubal endothelium), creating a hostile environment for the transport of the fertilized egg and promoting an increased risk for a tubal (ectopic) pregnancy.

Other factors that have been implicated as causes of first trimester losses include autoimmune disorders such as the antiphospholipid antibody syndromes, substance abuse, cigarette smoking, multiple pregnancies, and placental abnormalities such as gestational trophoblastic diseases, the most common being molar pregnancies.

Treatments for imminent miscarriage or first trimester loss are unfortunately usually expectant. They have included strict bed rest and administeration of hormonal supplements as well as other exogenous therapies. In circumstances where there is a viable pregnancy and significant vaginal bleeding, bed rest may be beneficial to reduce trauma in an already precarious pregnancy. Such is the case with the vanishing twin syndrome, where conception resulted in a twin gestation but one twin aborts, causing bleeding, while the remaining twin is viable. Progesterone therapy is thought to be of value in circumstances where there might be reduced progesterone production from the ovary, leading to poor embryonic development (inadequate luteal phase). Aspirin, steroids such as prednisone, and heparin have been used with some success in the treatment of immunological causes of pregnancy loss.

Genetic Disorders

Michael R. Berman, MD

The second trimester begins at about 13 weeks and continues until the 27th week. This trimester is unique in that it spans a time period where a previable fetus becomes a potentially viable neonate, albeit premature (preterm). At exactly what week or day or fetal/neonatal weight this transformation occurs depends on many factors and unknowns. In current practice (1995) it is generally felt that a birth prior to 24 weeks is unlikely to survive, although it is not impossible and without hope. (When I was an ob-gyn resident in 1973, 28 weeks was considered the critical gestational age.) Losses in the third trimester have etiologies similar to those of the second trimester.

Chromosomal abnormalities account for nearly 15% of second-trimester pregnancy losses. Fortunately, pregnant women have an opportunity for a comprehensive prenatal evaluation of their fetus to determine genetic and morphologic (structural) normaly. Although it is not mandatory, women at risk for fetal problems may avail themselves of several testing procedures and may be offered screening procedures. Because some tests are invasive (e.g., amniocentesis, chorionic villus sampling [CVS], fetal blood sampling, and direct fetal visualization [fetoscopy]), it is important for the patient and her physician to have a clear understanding of what information is to be ascertained from a particular test, and the test's risks and limitations. Other tests, such as blood screening and high-resolution ultrasound, are less invasive. With these guidelines well defined, the prenatal diagnosis of fetal abnormalities becomes an important tool in the care of pregnancy.

Prepregnancy counseling is very important, and women should consult their physician or other primary caregiver prior to conception, or at least very early in the first trimester, so as to determine any risk factors for genetic diseases (e.g., familial disorders such as cystic fibrosis, muscular dystrophy, hemophilia, sickle cell anemia, and Tay-Sachs disease, or chromosomal disorders, the most common being Down syndrome or trisomy 21). Carrier states can then be detected prior to conception or early in the pregnancy. Appropriate diagnostic tools may be utilized as described above: blood sampling, CVS, amniocentesis, and high-resolution ultrasound. For families who have been identified at risk for hereditary diseases, genetic counseling is indicated. Genetic centers are usually integrated into university centers.

For families not at risk for genetic disorders, certain screening tests (noninvasive) are available. The maternal alpha-fetoprotein (AFP) test (now combined with two other markers, human chorionic gonadotropin and estriol) screens primarily for two particular classes of disorders: neural tube defects and chromosome abnormalities, the most common being Down syndrome or trisomy 21). If the test results is positive, either above or below the limits of the mean, it does not necessarily indicate that there *is* a problem—only that there might be a higher risk of a problem. The next procedural step is to perform a detailed ultrasound exam, sometimes called a "level 2" scan, and possibly an amniocentesis. These second-line tests can better define the health of the fetus within the limitations of each.

Genetic testing, although available for many years, is on the cusp of a new frontier—that of very early, embryonic diagnosis via microfetal blood sampling and maternal blood sampling for fetal cells and fetal chromosome analysis. Early fetal treatment may also be possible through gene manipulation and therapy.

Genetically abnormal embryos that develop and survive the first trimester can be diagnosed by prenatal tests, or be manifested by spontaneous labor or intrauterine fetal demise. One example of an abnormal chromosomal arrangement, which presents with premature rupture of the fetal membranes, premature labor, or fetal demise is trisomy 18. Although this can be detected by CVS, amniocentesis, and/or ultrasound, most patients not at risk will not have these procedures. Maternal serum AFP testing can screen low-risk populations, but, because it is only a screening tool, some patients may not avail themselves of it and others may have a false negative report. Trisomy 18 is not compatible with life, and early diagnosis can offer affected parents the option for elective termination.

Voluntary termination of a genetically abnormal fetus in the second trimester is no less anguishing than spontaneous previable miscarriage or delivery, for it involves not only loss but also conscious decision making at a time when one's mind is filled with remorse. Patients at this time need caring and informative counseling to help with their decision-making process. If at all possible, counseling with a geneticist is the ideal. As difficult as the decisions associated with situations of fetal death or nonviability are, diagnoses involving anomalous chromosomes or handicapping physical abnormalities in a fetus who will be born alive and survive are even more difficult. It is not my intention here to be judgmental or to express opinions about the ethics of any options a physician might offer a patient facing these onerous problems. All options must be discussed and offered in an atmosphere of information, compassion, and objectivity.

The Incompetent Cervix

Michael R. Berman, MD

With advancing fetal age, the expanding volume of the uterus places increasing forces upon the cervix. In the normal pregnancy, the cervix maintains significant strength to resist this pressure, which can lead to dilation and effacement in the second and early third trimesters. Certain conditions predispose the cervix to premature dilation and effacement, which can lead to premature labor and pregnancy loss. When either condition occurs, it is presumed to be a consequence of weakened cervical tissue fibers and has therefore been called "the incompetent cervix." The incompetent cervix accounts for approximately 15% of all second trimester losses. The most common etiologies or predisposing factors for an incompetent cervix are

1. Maternal diethylstilbestrol (DES) exposure;
2. Prior conization (biopsy of the cervix);
3. Repeated dilation of the cervix;
4. Traumatic injury to the cervix.

DES is a synthetic estrogen that was given to women in the 1950s and 1960s to prevent repeated miscarriages. It was discovered in the early 1970s that as they entered their teenage years, the daughters of these women were developing abnormalities of the cervix called adenosis and, rarely, adenocarcinoma (cancer) of the vagina—an extremely rare form of cancer. Although most of the changes are benign, women with adenosis have a higher incidence of infertility and miscarriage, particularly in the second trimester. The adenosis that affects the morphology of the cervix weakens it, resulting in an incompetent cervix. Most women exposed to DES do not have this problem, but the history of DES exposure is so very important that pregnant "DES daughters" should be followed more closely.

Conization of the cervix is a procedure that is performed to diagnose and treat cancerous or precancerous changes in the cervix. A large portion of the cervix that contains the abnormal (dysplastic) cells is excised, and, along with it, almost invariably, a portion of the muscle and connective tissue of the cervix, which contributes to its weakening. Newer techniques, such as laser therapy and electrical loop excision therapy, can theoretically reduce the amount of tissue destruction, but should still be taken into consideration.

Patients who have undergone multiple therapeutic abortions and dilation of the cervix are at increased risk for an incompetent cervix because the muscle and connective tissue of the cervix can lose their elasticity and remain stretched if dilation with mechanical dilators is performed multiple times. The appropriate treatment for these patients is frequent examinations in the second trimester.

The diagnosis of incompetent cervix is not an exact methodology. Examinations early in the second trimester are important for any women with a history of any of the above factors or any women with a history of an unexplained second trimester loss, particularly if it occurred without much pain or bleeding—the "silent dilation of the cervix." Early diagnosis of premature dilation of the cervix can lead to therapy that can sustain the pregnancy to and beyond the threshold of viability. Ultrasound examinations looking for endocervical length, funneling, dilation, and effacement are helpful, and the parameter of shortened endocervical length is most predictive. Should the cervix be found to be dilated or particularly thinned (effaced), a suture can be placed around the cervix and tied to give it strength. This is called a cervical cerclage. The two most utilized techniques for cervical cerclage are the Shirodkar and the McDonald procedures. They yield similar results, and their use depends mostly on the training and experience of the operating surgeon. The premise for the cerclage is to further close the cervix and reinforce the connective tissue with high tensile-strength suture, so as to maintain the integrity of the pregnancy. The procedure is most commonly performed just after the first trimester and can be done on an outpatient basis under regional (spinal or epidural) or general anesthesia. Although this provides strength to the weakened cervix, the therapy for incompetent cervix must also include bed rest, sometimes throughout the pregnancy; possible use of tocolysis (stopping labor with medications); and hospitalization when needed. In the appropriately selected population, cervical cerclage can be very effective and yields an excellent prognosis for term or near-term delivery.

The Antiphospholipid Antibody Syndrome

Sara Marder, MD

Many causes have been linked to recurrent pregnancy loss. One of the less frequently seen associations is the antiphospholipid antibody syndrome.

WHAT ARE ANTIPHOSPHOLIPID ANTIBODIES?

Under normal circumstances, antibodies are proteins made by the immune system to fight substances recognized as foreign by the body. Examples of foreign substances are bacteria and viruses. Sometimes the body's own cells are recognized as foreign. In the antiphospholipid antibody syndrome the body recognizes phospholipids (part of a cell's membrane) as foreign and produces antibodies against them. Antibodies to phospholipids (antiphospholipid antibodies) can be found in the blood of some people with lupus, but they are also seen in people without any known illness. Lupus anticoagulant (LAC) and anticardiolipin antibody (ACA) are the two known antiphospholipid antibodies that are associated with recurrent pregnancy loss.

WHAT IS THE ANTIPHOSPHOLIPID ANTIBODY SYNDROME?

Different physicians may use slightly different definitions to diagnose the antiphospholipid antibody syndrome. In general, you must have a positive blood test for either LAC or ACA on two separate occasions, at least eight weeks apart. In addition to the blood tests you must have one the following: a history of thrombosis (clots within the blood vessels), thrombocytopenia (low platelet count), or recurrent pregnancy loss. Other manifestations that may be seen in patients with the antiphospholipid antibody syndrome include skin, heart, and nervous system abnormalities.

WHAT IS THE ASSOCIATION BETWEEN ANTIPHOSPHOLIPID ANTIBODIES AND PREGNANCY LOSS?

Among women with recurrent pregnancy losses, antiphospholipid antibodies have been reported in 11%–22%. LAC and/or medium-to-high ACA have been associated with first, second, and third trimester pregnancy losses. The association is even higher when the antiphospholipid antibody tests are persistently positive. Although it is unknown exactly how the antiphospholipid antibody syndrome adversely affects pregnancy, one theory is that it may cause blood clots. These blood clots, which can be microscopic, may occur in the blood vessels of the placenta. The placenta provides nourishment to the baby, and any interruption in this process can be harmful to the pregnancy. The antiphospholipid antibody syndrome may increase the risk of miscarriage, poor fetal growth, preeclampsia (high blood pressure during pregnancy), and stillbirth. It has yet to be proved, but many researchers think the antiphospholipid antibody syndrome may exist in a state of remission or exacerbation similar to diseases such as lupus and rheumatoid arthritis. This means there can be periods when the antibodies are not active.

WHO SHOULD BE TESTED FOR ANTIPHOSPHOLIPID ANTIBODY SYNDROME?

Women who have had a history of recurrent pregnancy losses should be tested for antiphospholipid antibodies. A history of unexplained poor fetal growth and or the early onset of severe preeclampsia or an unexplained placental abruption is an indication for testing. A history of thrombosis, stroke, heart attack, thrombocytopenia (low platelet count), presence of other autoimmune disorders such as lupus, an abnormal venereal disease research laboratory test or partial prothrombin time blood test would suggest the need for testing.

WHAT IS THE TREATMENT FOR THE ANTIPHOSPHOLIPID ANTIBODY SYNDROME IN PREGNANCY?

The drug of choice for treatment is heparin, which is injected to prevent blood from clotting. It is used in combination with "baby" (low dose) aspirin. In certain cases prednisone and baby aspirin are used to treat the antiphospholipid antibody syndrome. All medications have side effects, and the choice of therapy should be made after the risks and benefits of the treatments have been discussed by the physician and the patient. These pregnancies should be monitored closely by ultrasound every month, to check on fetal growth, and by antenatal testing (nonstress tests and biophysical profiles) weekly, beginning at 32 weeks' gestation. Although there are a few reports of successful pregnancies without treatment, the majority of researchers have reported a 70%–75% success rate with treatment.

Preimplantation Genetic Diagnosis

Anuja Dokras, MD, PhD

With recent advances in genetics, several inherited disorders can now be diagnosed at a molecular level. For couples who are carriers or are affected by any of these conditions and are at high risk for transmitting it to their offspring, it is possible to detect the disorder during pregnancy. This is done by one of two approaches: amniocentesis or chorionic villus sampling (which involves taking a small sample of the placenta at an early stage). The couples then face the dilemma of whether or not to terminate the pregnancy if the genetic abnormality is present. In some cases this may not be a viable option for religious or moral reasons. An alternative would then be to diagnose the condition in the embryo stage, before the pregnancy is established. Only the unaffected embryos would then be transferred to the uterus. This technique, referred to as preimplantation genetic diagnosis, would obviate the need for screening during a pregnancy and hence prevent the physical and psychological trauma associated with termination.

HOW CAN A DIAGNOSIS BE MADE IN THE PREIMPLANTATION PERIOD?

Research toward developing techniques for early genetic diagnosis in humans was initiated in the United Kingdom in the late 1980s.[1] In vitro fertilization (IVF) techniques are used to obtain eggs from the mother, which are then fertilized in the laboratory with sperm obtained from the father. One or more cells are removed from the developing embryo two to four days after fertilization. This highly sophisticated technique, called micromanipulation, does not adversely affect further development of the embryo. The cells removed are analyzed, and the results can be obtained within twelve to twenty four hours. The embryos without the genetic defects are transferred into the uterus to develop into a normal pregnancy.

WHAT CONDITIONS CAN BE SCREENED?

Almost all genetically inherited conditions that are diagnosed in the prenatal period can be detected in the preimplantation period. Diseases that have a high risk of transmission (25%–50%) and are usually associated with significant morbidity and mortality can be screened for by this technique. The limiting factor is that few cells (usually only one to two) are available for diagnosis, in contrast to amniocentesis or CVS. Therefore obtaining an accurate diagnosis requires laboratory tests prior to the clinical application of this technique for a given disease.

HAVE BABIES BEEN BORN AFTER APPLICATION OF THIS TECHNIQUE?

The first report of the successful application of this technique came from the Hammersmith Hospital, London, which currently is the center with the highest number of births following preimplantation diagnosis. Over thirty such pregnancies have now been reported worldwide. The conditions screened for include cystic fibrosis, Tay-Sachs disease, hemophilia, fragile X syndrome, and rarer conditions such as Bart's syndrome and Rett's syndrome.

WHY DOES THE TECHNIQUE INVOLVE IVF?

Currently IVF is the only available method for obtaining an embryo in the very early stages of development. Therefore, although couples with a high risk of transmitting a genetic defect to their offspring may have normal fertility, they need to go through the IVF procedure to provide embryos for screening. Not surprisingly, the pregnancy rate in this group has been shown to be higher than that in patients with documented infertility.

TO WHOM WOULD THIS APPROACH BE APPLICABLE?

This technique is currently available to couples whose offspring are at a high risk (25%–50%) for a specific genetic condition because one or both parents are carriers or are affected by the disease. Also, the genetic code associated with the condition must be known in order to allow diagnosis. Currently it is not feasible to routinely screen women at lower risks, such as women over age thirty-five for Down syndrome, since the pregnancy is established through IVF.

WHAT NEXT?

Only a few centers offer preimplantation diagnosis to couples at high risk or those who already have an affected child. Efforts continue to be focused on improving methods to obtain an accurate diagnosis from only one or two cells. Techniques are now available to screen for more than one condition simultaneously, but the accuracy of these modifications needs to be tested further. Although there is certainly a demand for this approach, it will continue to be available only in specialized institutions with excellent IVF and molecular biology laboratories.

Congenital Heart Disease

Joshua A. Copel, MD

Congenital heart disease is one of the most common congenital anomalies. Overall, approximately 3% of newborns have some major congenital anomaly, and about 15% of these have congenital heart disease. Looked at another way, about 30,000 infants die annually in the United States between 5 months' pregnancy and one year after birth. One in five die because of congenital anomalies, and one in three of these are cardiovascular abnormalities.

The origin of cardiac abnormalities lies in the complex development of the heart. Starting out as a single straight, hollow tube, the heart must divide into two sides, and fold over on itself twice to begin to reach its final form. Some areas must differentiate into electrical conduction tissues, and others into muscle, and still others must develop into the strong tissues of the valves that keep blood moving in the proper direction. When one considers the incredible complexity of this process, it becomes easier to understand that there are many ways in which the heart can develop abnormally. The most common fetal cardiac abnormalities are complete atrioventricular septal defect ("canal" defect), hypoplastic left heart syndrome, and double outlet right ventricle/tetralogy of Fallot. Other abnormalities are much less common than these three (the third involves a spectrum of abnormalities that are all related etiologically). In newborns the most common defect is atrioventricular septal defect.

Newborns with congenital heart disease usually look much like unaffected newborns for the first few hours after birth. Before birth the heart is specially adapted for intrauterine life. The fetus does not breathe inside the womb; the placenta does the breathing for it. Normally there are connections between the right and left receiving chambers of the heart (the atria) and between the two main arteries that leave the heart: the aorta, to the body, and the pulmonary artery, to the lungs.

Newborns with many types of severe heart problems do well until these normal connections begin the process of closing. At that point, fetuses lacking one of the normal pumping chambers—a ventricle, for example—begin to show the abnormal coloration or labored breathing that is often the first sign of cardiac abnormalities. These signs are similar to those seen in newborns with infections and some other problems, so it may take a couple of hours to recognize that a heart problem is present. Especially in these days of early hospital discharges for apparently healthy moms and babies, problems may not arise until the child has been brought home. For parents of a first child, recognizing that there is a problem can take a while.

Certain groups of pregnant women have been identified as being at special risk for delivering a baby with a heart abnormality. Women who have had a child with heart disease have a 2%–3% risk of having another (1 in 30–50). If the mother was born with a heart abnormality, the risk may be as high as 5% (1 in 20). Some medications, such as those used to control epilepsy, can damage the baby's developing heart, but are important for the mother to take for her own health. Recently, high doses of Vitamin A (10,000 units a day or more) have been identified as causing a high risk of fetal heart abnormalities. Oral contraceptives and fertility medications, such as Clomid® and Pergonal®, appear to be safe.

It is fortunate that testing is available for pregnancies identified as being at high risk for fetal heart abnormalities. A fetal echocardiogram uses the same ultrasound technology that is used for measuring the fetus and taking pictures of other parts of the fetus. In a fetal echocardiogram the entire heart is systematically examined for normal development. Any areas of suspected abnormality can be evaluated in detail, often by using special ultrasound techniques, called Doppler ultrasound, that measure the direction and speed of blood as it flows through the heart. Fetal echocardiograms should be performed by physicians with special expertise in the examination of the fetal heart. These may be obstetricians, pediatric cardiologists, or radiologists, usually working in a team effort. Echocardiograms showing suspected abnormalities are generally referred to regional or supraregional centers with extensive experience in evaluating the test.

What if a fetal heart abnormality is found? The first step is to perform a thorough examination of the rest of the fetal anatomy, to be sure that no other abnormalities are present that might complicate caring for the newborn. Next comes consultation with a pediatric cardiologist to discuss what might need to be done for the newborn. This usually includes discussion of delivery at a pediatric heart center where the baby can be operated on if necessary. It is especially important psychologically for the parents to be near the baby. The operations that may need to be done are discussed, and the long-term outlook for the baby can be outlined. If the pregnancy is early enough, and the long-term outlook is bleak, many families choose to terminate the pregnancy, an unpleasant alternative but an important choice to include in discussions with the parents. Delivery is usually vaginal; there is no evidence that cardiac babies do better if delivered by cesarean section.

Being prepared with knowledge of the presence of a heart abnormality, the pediatric team can plan for the delivery. We find it helpful for the parents to meet with the hospital neonatal intensive care specialists beforehand and to tour the nursery to familiarize themselves with where their baby will be and the people who will be taking care of it.

Placental Causes of Fetal Loss

David Lima, MD

The word "placenta" was introduced in 1691 and is derived from the Latin word for "flat cake." The placenta or afterbirth is the organ of metabolic exchange between the fetus and the mother. It has a portion derived from the developing embryo and a maternal portion formed by modification of the uterine lining. There is no direct mixing of fetal and maternal blood. The intervening tissue is sufficiently thin to permit the entry of nutrients and oxygen into the fetal blood and the release of carbon dioxide and waste materials from it. In the third trimester of pregnancy the placenta is a disk-shaped organ approximately 20 centimeters (cm) across and 2 to 3 cm thick. It has a maternal surface, attached to the uterus, and a fetal surface. The umbilical cord extends from the fetus to the fetal surface of the placenta. There are six abnormalities of the placenta that can result in fetal death:

1. Placental abruption
2. Trauma
3. Circulatory disturbances
4. Abnormalities of placentation
5. Tumors of the placenta
6. Abnormalities of the umbilical cord.

PLACENTAL ABRUPTION

Placental abruption is defined as separation of the maternal surface of the placenta from the uterus before delivery of the fetus. It occurs in approximately 0.9% of pregnancies and accounts for 15% to 25% of all perinatal mortality (stillbirths and neonatal deaths). Placental abruption often occurs without advance notice. Its most common symptom is painful vaginal bleeding, but the clinical presentation is variable. Some of the bleeding of placental abruption usually escapes through the cervix, resulting in recognizable external hemorrhage. Less commonly, the blood is retained between the detached maternal surface of the placenta and the uterus, resulting in a concealed hemorrhage. Although abruptions may occur at any time during a pregnancy, approximately 42% occur after 37 weeks (term). The primary cause of placental abruption is unknown, but there are several associated conditions, including maternal hypertension (both pregnancy-induced and chronic), cigarette smoking, cocaine use, advanced maternal age, increasing parity (number of births), abdominal trauma (especially motor vehicle accidents), and preterm premature rupture of the membranes. Placental abruption may be total or partial. Treatment for it varies, depending upon the condition of the mother and the fetus. If there is significant bleeding, blood transfusions and prompt delivery may be lifesaving for the mother and the fetus. If the mother is stable and the fetus is immature (preterm) and not compromised, expectant management with very close observation and continuous electronic fetal heart rate monitoring in a hospital may be beneficial. However, facilities and personnel for immediate intervention must be available. The risk of recurrent abruption in a subsequent pregnancy is high, approximately 12%. The frequency of placental abruption fatal to the fetus has declined to about 1 in 800 deliveries.

TRAUMA

Trauma and accidents are the leading cause of death in young reproductive-age women. It is estimated that 1 in 12 pregnancies will be complicated by trauma. Motor vehicle accidents are the most common cause of blunt trauma to the pregnant woman. The use of seat belts with shoulder straps is recommended at all times. Other causes of trauma include falls and, unfortunately, assaults, which appear to be increasing in frequency. Traumatic placental abruption reportedly complicates 1% to 6% of "minor" injuries and up to 50% of major injuries. Placental abruption usually develops soon after trauma. In the absence of placental abruption, fetal injury and death are uncommon. If the placenta is lacerated, fetal blood may hemorrhage into the maternal circulation.

CIRCULATORY DISTURBANCES

"Infarction" or "infarct" refers to an area of cell death and tissue necrosis resulting from insufficient blood supply. Microscopic thrombi (blood clots) may form within blood vessels, impeding blood flow, and are a common cause of infarction. This is usually what occurs during a heart attack (myocardial infarction) secondary to occlusion of a coronary artery. Constriction or closure of blood vessels (vasoconstriction) can occur for a variety of reasons, most commonly as a result of hypertension. Additionally, certain substances, such as cocaine, are vasoactive and are known to cause closure of blood vessels and subsequent infarction. The placenta is a highly vascular organ. Any process that adversely affects blood vessels can damage placental blood vessels as well as the uterine blood vessels (spiral arteries) that feed the placenta. Placental infarcts are common features of a normal "aging" placenta. They are found in approximately 25% of uncomplicated term pregnancies and appear to be of no clinical significance. However, certain maternal diseases, such as severe hypertension and connective tissue disorders (e.g., lupus, antiphospholipid antibody syndrome, scleroderma, and rheumatoid arthritis) may lead to extensive placental infarction. If the placenta is partially compromised (uteroplacental insufficiency), the fetus may not be able to grow appropriately (intrauterine growth restriction—IUGR). In severe cases, blood flow to and from the placenta may not be enough to keep the fetus alive.

ABNORMALITIES OF PLACENTATION

When the placenta is located over or very near the internal opening (os) of the cervix, it is termed placenta previa. Placenta previa is classified as marginal, partial, or total, depending on the relationship of the placenta to the internal opening of the cervix (e.g., a total placenta previa completely covers the cervix). Placenta previa occurs when the zygote implants very low in the uterus, close to the internal cervical opening. These placentas usually "migrate" away from the cervix as the pregnancy progresses and the uterus increases in size to accommodate the growing fetus. Placenta previa complicates approximately 1 in 200 deliveries. The most common presentation is painless vaginal bleeding in the third trimester. The major complications of placenta previa are maternal hemorrhage and shock and significant perinatal mortality (stillbirths and neonatal deaths). Although approximately half of patients are near term when bleeding first develops, preterm delivery remains a major cause of perinatal death. The primary cause of placenta previa is unknown, but there are several risk factors, including advanced maternal age, high parity (number of births), prior cesarean section, prior elective abortion, multiple fetuses, and cigarette smoking. Placenta previa may be associated with abnormal attachment of the placenta to the uterus (placenta accreta, increta, or percreta), especially if the placenta previa is located over a previous cesarean section scar. As with placental abruption, the treatment of placenta previa varies, depending upon the condition of the mother and the fetus.

TUMORS OF THE PLACENTA

Tumors may develop in the placenta. Chorioangiomas, the most common type of placental tumor, are benign hemangiomas of the fetal blood vessels. They have been reported in approximately 1% of placentas. Small tumors are usually asymptomatic and of no clinical significance. However, large tumors (greater than 5 cm in diameter) may be associated with polyhydramnios (too much amniotic fluid) and premature labor, or antepartum hemorrhage. Fetal death and malformations are uncommon complications. Metastases of malignant tumors to the placenta are exceedingly rare. Malignant melanoma is reportedly the most common malignancy metastatic to the placenta (others include leukemia and lymphomas). Gestational trophoblastic disease refers to a spectrum of pregnancy-related placental trophoblast growth abnormalities. Briefly, gestational trophoblastic disease can be divided into hydatidiform moles (complete and partial molar pregnancy) and gestational trophoblastic tumors (invasive mole, choriocarcinoma, and placental-site tumor). Complete moles do not contain a fetus. The fetus of a partial mole is not viable. Hydatidiform moles (complete and partial) tend to present as incomplete or threatened abortions (miscarriage). Rarely two placentas may coexist, with a hydatidiform mole developing alongside a normal-appearing placenta and its fetus. Gestational trophoblastic tumors almost always develop with or follow some form of pregnancy (normal, molar, and ectopic pregnancy, miscarriage, or elective abortion). Malignancy is rarely identified in the placenta of a normal-appearing pregnancy, but may follow an otherwise normal pregnancy. With prompt treatment by experienced physicians specializing in these tumors, the prognosis and cure rates are excellent.

ABNORMALITIES OF THE UMBILICAL CORD

Abnormalities of Cord Length

Umbilical cord length varies considerably. The average length is approximately 55 cm. Abnormal extremes of cord length range from apparently no cord (achordia) to up to 300 cm. Vascular occlusion by thrombi (blood clots) and true knots are more common in excessively long cords. Long cords are also more likely to prolapse through the cervix prior to delivery of the fetus. Cord prolapse is more common when the fetus is small (e.g., preterm deliveries) and in certain types of breech presentations (e.g., footling breech). Cord prolapse impairs blood flow to the fetus and requires immediate delivery by cesarean section. Fortunately, the incidence of cord prolapse is relatively low, complicating approximately 0.5% of all births. Footling breech presentations are typically delivered by elective cesarean section to prevent this and other potential complications of vaginal delivery. Rarely, abnormally short umbilical cords may rupture or cause placental abruption.

Abnormalities of Cord Insertion

The umbilical cord usually inserts near the center of the fetal surface of the placenta. The blood vessels in the umbilical cord are protected by a jellylike substance (Wharton's jelly). In certain instances, the umbilical cord inserts at a distance from the placenta, and its blood vessels must travel relatively unprotected in the fetal membranes to reach the placenta. This condition is termed velamentous insertion of the umbilical cord and occurs in approximately 1% of pregnancies; it is more frequent with twins and triplets. Rarely, these unprotected vessels may rupture and result in fetal death from hemorrhage. Additionally, with velamentous insertion of the umbilical cord, some of the blood vessels may cross the cervix, a condition termed vasa previa. With vasa previa, rupture of the fetal membranes ("breaking the water"), either spontaneously or by the obstetrician/nurse-midwife (amniotomy), may be accompanied by rupture of a fetal blood vessel, which can result in fetal death from hemorrhage. The amount of blood loss sufficient to kill the fetus is relatively small. In contrast, hemorrhage from placental abruption is blood lost from the mother, and a much larger hemorrhage may be associated with a good outcome for the mother and fetus.

Absence of One Umbilical Artery

The umbilical cord normally contains three blood vessels (one vein and two arteries). Two vessel cords, with only one artery, are found in less than 1% of pregnancies (more common in twins and in fetuses of mothers with diabetes). Approximately 30% of all fetuses with two vessel cords have associated congenital anomalies. Additionally, fetuses with two vessel cords have a higher incidence of IUGR, preterm delivery, and miscarriage (spontaneous abortion).

Cord Abnormalities

Several abnormalities of the umbilical cord are capable of impairing blood flow between the placenta and the fetus. True knots are thought to result from active fetal movements and are found in approximately 1% of pregnancies. Fetal death may result in approximately 6% of pregnancies complicated by true knots. The incidence of true knots may be increased with an abnormally long umbilical cord and is especially high in monoamniotic twins. Loops of umbilical cord frequently become coiled around the fetus, most commonly the neck (nuchal cord). Fortunately, nuchal cords are an uncommon cause of fetal death. The umbilical cord normally becomes twisted as a result of fetal movements (torsion of the cord). Rarely, twisting of the cord on itself is so severe that blood flow is compromised, resulting in fetal death. In monoamniotic twins, with no fetal membrane separating the fetuses, the two umbilical cords may become twisted around each other. Rarely, hematomas of the umbilical cord result from rupture of one of the umbilical blood vessels, usually the vein. Cysts of the umbilical cord may form but rarely are clinically significant. These "cord accidents" are rare causes of fetal death, and it is probably unwise to attribute fetal death to a cord accident until other causes have been ruled out.

Behind Every Healthy Baby Is a Healthy Placenta

Harvey J. Kliman, MD, PhD

The placenta is the single most important factor in producing a healthy baby. It is in fact part of the fetus and thus is critical for all aspects of pregnancy from implantation to delivery. As early as three days after fertilization, the trophoblasts, the major cell type of the placenta, begin to make human chorionic gonadotropin, a hormone that ensures that the endometrium will be receptive to the implanting embryo. Over the next few days, these trophoblasts attach to and invade the uterine lining, beginning the process of pregnancy. Over the next few weeks the placenta begins to make hormones that control the basic physiology of the mother in such a way that the fetus is supplied with the nutrients and oxygen needed for successful growth. The placenta also protects the fetus from immune attack by the mother, removes waste products from the fetus, induces the mother to bring more blood to the placenta, and, near the time of delivery, produces hormones that mature the fetal organs in preparation for life outside of the uterus. In many ways the placenta is the SCUBA system for the fetus and at the same time is the Houston Control Center guiding the mother through pregnancy. The placenta is dedicated to the survival of the fetus. Even when exposed to a poor maternal environment—for example, when the mother is malnourished or diseased, smokes, or takes cocaine—the placenta can often compensate by becoming more efficient. However, there are limits to the placenta's ability to cope with external stresses. Eventually, if multiple or severe enough, these stresses can lead to placental damage, fetal damage, and even intrauterine demise and pregnancy loss.

Just as the rings of a cut tree can tell the story of the tree's life, so the placenta can disclose the history of the pregnancy. In cases of poor pregnancy outcome, microscopic examination of the placenta often reveals the stresses that caused the fetal damage observed in an affected newborn.

The major pathologic processes observable in the placenta that can adversely affect pregnancy outcome include intrauterine bacterial infections, decreased blood flow to the placenta from the mother, and attack on the placenta by the mother's immune system. Intrauterine infections, most commonly the result of migration of vaginal bacteria through the cervix into the uterine cavity, can lead to severe fetal hypoxia as a result of villous edema (fluid buildup within the placenta). Both chronic and acute decreases in blood flow to the placenta can cause severe fetal damage and even death. Besides supplying the fetus with nutrition, the placenta is a barrier between the mother and the fetus, protecting the fetus from immune rejection by the mother, a pathologic process that can lead to intrauterine growth retardation or even demise. In addition to these major pathologic categories, many other insults, such as placental separation, cord accidents, trauma, and viral and parasitic infections, can adversely affect pregnancy outcome by affecting the function of the placenta.

A trained placental pathologist can examine a placenta and assist in the elucidation of the causes of poor pregnancy outcome. A complete placental examination is most useful shortly after delivery, when the affected family most needs to understand what happened to their baby. If a full placental examination is not possible because no placental pathologist is available, the placenta can be transferred to a center that is prepared to make such an examination. As long as tissue blocks are saved from the placenta, a microscopic examination of the placenta is possible at a later time if the need arises.

Today, only a few specialized centers for placental examination exist in the United States. As the cost of processing and examining placentas decreases, more of the 4 million placentas delivered every year will be able to be examined by appropriately trained physicians. This trend will lead to a better understanding of causes of poor pregnancy outcomes, which in turn will lead to better diagnostic and therapeutic approaches to complicated pregnancies. The ultimate goal of placental examination and research is to ensure that wanted babies are healthy babies.

Intrauterine Growth Restriction

Giancarlo Mari, MD

DEFINITION OF IUGR

"Intrauterine growth restriction" (IUGR) is the most common generic term used to describe the fetus with a birth weight at or below the tenth percentile for gestational age and sex. This term is often erroneously used as a synonym for small for gestational age (SGA). The IUGR fetus does not reach its potential of growth, whereas the SGA fetus does. In other words, a fetus with a potential of growth at the fiftieth percentile but, because of maternal, fetal, or placental disorders occurring alone or in combination, becomes growth restricted (birthweight < tenth percentile) is an IUGR fetus and is at risk for adverse perinatal outcome. A fetus with a potential of growth at the seventh percentile that reaches its potential of growth (seventh percentile) is not an IUGR fetus but an SGA fetus. It is a normal small fetus and is not at risk for adverse perinatal outcome.

The two components that are necessary to define an IUGR fetus are

a. Birthweight < tenth percentile
b. Pathologic process that inhibits expression of the normal intrinsic growth potential.

The two components that are necessary to define an SGA fetus are

a. Birthweight < tenth percentile
b. Absence of pathologic process.

INCIDENCE

The incidence of SGA fetuses in the population is approximately 7%; 10%–15% of SGA fetuses are IUGR fetuses.

ETIOLOGY

Both maternal and paternal race have a measurable effect on the fetal size and, therefore, an indirect effect on the incidence of SGA. These racial influences can have an impact on clinical practice. The application of a fetal growth curve derived from one population to a different population can result in over- or underestimation of the true incidence of SGA. Birth weight

132

and fetal growth rates tend to be least among populations of Asian extraction and greatest in populations of Nordic extraction. These racial differences can be quite dramatic, and at term the mean birth weight may vary by as much as 1,400 grams. The lowest mean birth weight has been noted in Asia (New Guinea, Lumi tribe: mean birth weight = 2,400 g); the largest mean birth weight has been noted in the Caribbean (Anguilla: mean birth weight = 3,880 g).

IUGR may be considered the consequence of a disease process within one or more of the three compartments that sustain and regulate fetal growth: the uterus, the placenta, and the fetus.

DIAGNOSIS OF THE RISK OF IUGR

Pregnancies at risk for IUGR may be diagnosed on the basis of previous history (e.g., low fetal birth weight in earlier pregnancies), associated disorders (autoimmune diseases, high blood pressure, etc.), and toxic habits (smoking, etc). Previous history of IUGR is the most important risk factor. In pregnancies with an increased risk, fetal growth should be closely monitored.

DIAGNOSIS OF PRESUMED OR SUSPECTED IUGR

This is perhaps the most important and the most difficult diagnosis to make, since most of IUGR pregnancies are free of any associated conditions that would alert the obstetrician to the possibility of IUGR. The discrepancy between gestational age and the size of the uterus is the clearest sign of IUGR. Therefore, basic screening for IUGR should be done using serial symphysis fundal height (SFH), reserving ultrasound biometrical data for cases in which the SFH falls below the fifth percentile.

DIAGNOSIS OF PROBABLE IUGR

The diagnosis of IUGR is based on biometrical parameters recorded during ultrasound scanning. In order to reduce misreading to a minimum, gestational age should be precisely determined. The most used biometrical parameters are the biparietal diameter, head circumference, abdominal circumference, head/abdominal circumference ratio, length of femur and humerus, and estimated fetal weight.

FETAL HEMODYNAMICS

IUGR is in most cases secondary to uteroplacental insufficiency. Much of the understanding of this phenomenon is derived from animal research. However, the advent of pulsed and color Doppler ultrasonography has allowed us to obtain noninvasive hemodynamic measurements from several vascular beds of the uterine, placental, and fetal circulation in humans.

DOPPLER ULTRASOUND

Doppler ultrasound gives us information on the vascular resistance and, indirectly, on the blood flow. Three indices are considered relative to the vascular resistance: systolic/diastolic (S/D) ratio, resistance index (RI; systolic velocity − diastolic velocity/systolic velocity), and pulsatility index (systolic velocity − diastolic velocity/mean velocity).

UTERINE CIRCULATION

The main uterine artery is the most commonly analyzed vessel. In normal pregnancy the S/D ratio and RI values significantly decrease with advancing gestation until 24 to 26 weeks. In the absence of this physiologic decrease, a higher incidence of hypertensive diseases and/or IUGR has been widely documented.

UMBILICAL ARTERY

In the normal fetus, the pulsatility index decreases with advancing gestation. This reflects a decrease of the placental vascular resistance. In fetuses with IUGR there is an increase of the pulsatility index secondary to the decrease, absence, or reversal of end-diastolic flow. The changes of these waveforms are thought to indicate increased placental resistance. The absent or reversed end-diastolic flow is strongly associated with an abnormal course of pregnancy and a higher incidence of perinatal complications, compared to fetuses with IUGR that are characterized by the presence of end-diastolic flow.

UMBILICAL VEIN

The umbilical vein has a continuous pattern following the first trimester. The presence of umbilical vein pulsations is associated with an increased risk of adverse perinatal outcome.

DUCTUS VENOSUS

The presence of reversed flow in the ductus venosus is an ominous sign. Goncalves et al. observed five fetuses with reverse flow velocity waveforms at the ductus venosus, and all the fetuses died in utero.[2] In 18 other fetuses with abnormal umbilical and middle cerebral artery waveforms, but without reverse flow in the ductus venosus, no deaths occurred.

FETAL CEREBRAL CIRCULATION

The middle cerebral artery is the vessel of choice to assess the fetal cerebral circulation because it is easy to identify, has a high reproducibility, and provides information on the brain-sparing effect. Additionally, it can be studied easily with an angle of zero degrees between the ultrasound beam and the direction of blood flow; therefore, information on the true velocity of the blood flow can be obtained.

BRAIN-SPARING EFFECT

Animal and human experiments have shown that there is an increase in blood flow to the brain in the IUGR fetus. This increase can be evidenced by Doppler ultrasound of the middle cerebral artery. This effect has been called the "brain-sparing effect" and is demonstrated by a lower value of the pulsatility index. In IUGR fetuses with a pulsatility index below the normal range, there is a greater incidence of adverse perinatal outcome. The brain-sparing effect may be transient, as reported during prolonged hypoxemia in animal experiments, and the overstressed human fetus can also lose the brain-sparing effect. The disappearance of the brain-sparing effect is a very critical event for the fetus and appears to precede fetal death. Unfortunately, to demonstrate this concept, it is necessary to perform a longitudinal study on severely IUGR fetuses up to the point of fetal demise. This has been confirmed in a few fetuses in situations where obstetrical intervention was refused by the parents. If this information is confirmed on a larger number of fetuses, the study of the middle cerebral artery may have tremendous implications for determining the proper timing of delivery.

UTEROPLACENTAL INSUFFICIENCY

Based on my personal experience, several phases of uteroplacental insufficiency may reflect changes in fetal hemodynamics.

Severe Uteroplacental Insufficiency

The substrate for the development of uteroplacental insufficiency may be laid down as early as the time of implantation. However, no effect is seen on growth or Doppler until 20–24 weeks' gestation. These fetuses do not have signs of growth restriction or abnormal Doppler ultrasound prior to this time.

If the fetus is measurably small by ultrasound at 22–24 weeks' gestation, several Doppler patterns may occur.

1. The umbilical artery still has a normal pulsatility index (resistance index or S/D ratio); the middle cerebral artery has either a normal or an abnormal pulsatility index.

2. The umbilical artery has an abnormal pulsatility index; the middle cerebral artery has either a normal or an abnormal pulsatility index.

3. The umbilical artery and the middle cerebral artery both have an abnormal pulsatility index.

The fetus needs to be monitored very closely. Bed rest and oxygen therapy may be useful; however, if both vessels have an abnormal value at this early gestational age, it is very likely that the process will deteriorate and the chance of a delivery at term is remote.

The pulsatility index of the umbilical artery may increase and the pulsatility index of the middle cerebral artery may decrease. The other fetal vessels may still appear normal, with the only Doppler abnormalities the umbilical artery and middle cerebral artery. The fetus starts to show signs of IUGR. The biophysical profile is normal.

At this time the lack of fetal growth, and/or the development of pre-eclampsia/eclampsia, and/or a persistent abnormal biophysical profile may interrupt the process with delivery of the fetus. Such a fetus is at lower risk for the development of respiratory distress syndrome and intraventricular hemorrhage (IVH). We have reported that IUGR fetuses with brain-sparing effect are less likely to develop IVH. The reason is not completely understood. However, production of steroids as a result of stress may play an important role in this process.

If the fetus is not delivered, the process of continues. At this time tricuspid regurgitation may appear, and ductus venosus reverse flow and umbilical vein pulsations may be present intermittently. The biophysical profile may still appear normal.

When ductus venosus reverse flow and umbilical vein pulsations are present continuously, the fetus starts to lose the brain-sparing effect. The biophysical profile becomes abnormal. Fetal demise follows. The time interval between continuous presence of ductus venosus reverse flow and umbilical vein pulsations and fetal demise varies from six to twelve hours to two weeks. Oligohydramnios may be present at any stage of the above process.

This theory applies to a specific, common IUGR and not to fetuses with IUGR caused by smoking, placental abruption, or toxic drug exposure, which may have a different pathology.

Mild Uteroplacental Insufficiency

Uteroplacental insufficiency starts at or after implantation. However, no effect is seen on Doppler and growth until 26–32 weeks' gestation. The umbilical artery and the middle cerebral artery waveforms may be abnormal. However, the process is not severe enough to stop fetal growth completely or to cause deterioration. These cases may be followed with outpatient monitoring, and often deliver at term.

CONCLUSION

Fetuses with IUGR show evident modifications of Doppler parameters in the uteroplacental and fetal circulation. At present, the condition of fetuses with IUGR can accurately be assessed by sequential studies of Doppler waveforms from different vascular areas. There are, however, still many uncertainties concerning the relationships between the Doppler changes and the metabolic situation of the fetus—and, therefore, concerning the optimal timing of delivery to prevent an intrauterine injury.

Molar Pregnancy: Gestational Trophoblastic Disease

Adina Chelouche, MD

After fertilization the embryo differentiates into fetal and placental tissues. The fetal tissue develops into the baby and the placental tissue provides nourishment for the baby from the mother. During the first trimester, the placenta or trophoblast is many times larger than the fetus and has the ability to grow independently. The placenta may continue to grow even without a viable fetus present. In rarer cases, a molar pregnancy, abnormal placental tissue, can have the potential for uncontrolled growth, like a tumor. These tumors are also called gestational trophoblastic disease. Molar pregnancy, or hydatidiform mole, is a pregnancy that has defective growth patterns. The placental tissue grows abnormally, appearing as multiple cysts that have been classically described as a "bunch of grapes." There are two subtypes of moles: complete and partial. Complete moles have no fetal tissue present; partial moles have some fetal tissue and some normal placental tissue.

The chromosomal makeup of molar pregnancies is quite interesting. Complete moles arise from fertilization of an "empty egg" (an egg that has lost its genetic material). All the genetic material arises from the father by fertilization of either two sperm at once or of one sperm that duplicates its genes within the egg. A partial mole also has duplicate paternal genetic material, though the maternal chromosomal complement is intact. Therefore the genetic material is in triplicate.

Molar pregnancy is a clinical problem not only because it produces an abnormal pregnancy that in most cases needs to be terminated, but also because of its ability to have residual disease and, in severe cases, result in metastasis. The malignant form of the disease is called an invasive mole or choriocarcinoma.

EPIDEMIOLOGY

The incidence of molar pregnancy varies greatly by region, with a higher rate in Asian countries. In Taiwan the incidence is 1 in 125 live births; the incidence in the United States is 1 in 1,500. The main risk factor is advanced maternal age. Women over age forty have a fivefold to tenfold greater chance of molar pregnancy. Other possible risk factors are related to poor nutrition, particularly a low intake of carotene (vitamin A precursor). However, the association is poor.

REASONS FOR THE MOST COMMON PERINATAL LOSSES

SYMPTOMS AND SIGNS

Almost all patients with a complete molar pregnancy have vaginal bleeding in the first trimester. For the most part the symptoms mimic those of a miscarriage. Half of patients with a complete mole have uterine enlargement that is advanced for the gestational age. As is true in normal pregnancy, nausea and vomiting are common complaints. Toxemia, marked by high blood pressure, swelling, and protein in the uterine, which is for the most part limited to the third trimester, can be seen before 20 weeks in patients with a complete mole. A few patients can have findings of hyperthyroidism, such as a fast heartbeat, tremulousness, and feeling warm.

Patients with partial moles in general have fewer symptoms. They rarely have uterine enlargement, hyperthyroidism, or toxemia.

DIAGNOSIS

A complete molar pregnancy has characteristic findings on ultrasound. The placental tissue is swollen into cystlike structures and there is the absence of a fetus. A partial mole is hard to delineate from an early miscarriage in which the pregnancy is no longer viable. Another tool to help diagnose a molar pregnancy is the beta HCG levels. Beta HCG is a protein produced by the placenta that is used in pregnancy tests. It can be measured in both the urine and the blood. The blood test has the advantage of giving a quantitative level that corresponds to the gestational age of the pregnancy. In a complete mole the level of beta HCG can be abnormally high, >100,000 mIu/ml. A partial mole may have beta HCG levels in a high-to-normal range. More specific tests to delineate a molar pregnancy from an early pregnancy, which measure different subunits of the HCG protein, are being developed.

MANAGEMENT

Once the diagnosis of a molar pregnancy or a nonviable pregnancy suspicious for a partial mole is made, evacuation of the uterus is recommended with termination of the pregnancy. The products of conception are sent to pathology for a final diagnosis. A preoperative workup, such as a chest X-ray and liver function tests, should be performed to rule out any spread of the disease.

FOLLOW-UP

Because 20% of patients with a complete mole and 5%–7% with a partial mole may have residual disease, close follow-up is necessary. Beta HCG levels are monitored weekly until two normal values are obtained, and then monthly for six months. It is important for the patient to use contraception for six months so that rising HCG levels normal for pregnancy are not confused with residual disease. The birth control pill does not increase the risk of postmolar disease. After normal HCG values are obtained for six months, pregnancy is considered safe.

Persistent molar disease is assumed if the HCG levels plateau or rise, are still elevated six months after the termination of the pregnancy, or are >20,000 mIu/ml four weeks after the termination. If choriocarcinoma, a malignant form of the disease, is found on the pathology specimen, or if metastases are found on physical exam or chest X-ray, further treatment is necessary.

TREATMENT

Persistent disease is characterized as local or metastatic (spread to other organs). Metastatic disease is divided into two subgroups, called good prognosis and poor prognosis, based on how long the disease is present, the pretreatment beta HCG level, location of the spread, and whether prior chemotherapy failed. For local spread and good prognosis metastatic disease, the cornerstone of therapy is single-agent chemotherapy, such as methotrexate. This drug kills rapidly dividing cells and is used for treatment of early ectopic pregnancies as well. The cure rate for this low-risk group approaches 100%.

The treatment of poor prognosis metastatic disease is multiple chemotherapeutic agents. If brain metastases are found, local radiation therapy is needed. The cure rate for the poor prognosis group is more than 70%.

FUTURE FERTILITY

Fear of becoming pregnant after treatment for molar pregnancy is common. Most women can be assured that they will have a normal future pregnancy, though patients with a prior molar pregnancy have a 1%–2% risk of subsequent molar pregnancy. Early detection by ultrasound of a normal embryo and fetal heartbeat is important. Also, beta HCG levels should be followed after delivery. There is no increase in fetal anomalies in patients who were treated with chemotherapy for persistent molar disease.

Ectopic Pregnancy

Steven J. Fleischman, MD

Ovulation typically occurs two weeks into the menstrual cycle. The egg is released from the ovary and enters the end of the fallopian tube farthest from the uterus, the fimbriated end. Fertilization takes place in the fallopian tube close to the ovary. As the embryo develops within the first week, it moves down the fallopian tube and eventually implants into the wall of the uterus. This process occurs in more than 98% of pregnancies. An ectopic pregnancy, or tubal pregnancy, occurs when implantation of the embryo takes place anywhere outside of the uterus. The majority (>97%) of ectopic pregnancies are located in the fallopian tube. The remaining percentage occurs in the portion of the uterus where the fallopian tube enters (the cornu), in the ovary or the cervix, or even within the abdominal cavity outside the uterus. Another type of ectopic pregnancy is the heterotopic ectopic pregnancy, an ectopic pregnancy that coexists with an intrauterine pregnancy.

HOW COMMON IS AN ECTOPIC PREGNANCY, AND WHAT IS THE SIGNIFICANCE?

The past two decades in the United States have seen a marked increase in the number of ectopic pregnancies. In 1992 almost 2% of all pregnancies were ectopic, and ectopic pregnancy-related deaths accounted for 10% of all pregnancy-related deaths. The heterotopic ectopic pregnancy is rare and occurs at a rate of 1 in 7,000 pregnancies. Ectopic pregnancy remains the second leading cause of maternal mortality in the United States and is the leading cause of maternal mortality in the first trimester.

WHY DO ECTOPIC PREGNANCIES OCCUR?

There are many underlying problems that predispose women to having an ectopic pregnancy. In general there is a problem with the tube that does not permit the passage of the fertilized egg into the uterus. Some specific risk factors include the following:

1. History of infection of the tube. This may include pelvic inflammatory disease as well as other sexually transmitted diseases. The inflammation associated with the infection causes damage to the internal walls of the fallopian tube, narrowing the lumen.

2. Adhesions around the tube. Adhesions are bandlike pieces of tissue that can form

within the abdomen after surgery, infection, or endometriosis. These bands can cause a kinking of the fallopian tube and make passage of the embryo difficult.

3. Previous ectopic pregnancy. After having one ectopic pregnancy there is a 7%–15% risk of having another.

4. Developmental abnormalities of the tube. While rare, it is possible to have abnormalities of the fallopian tube. Women who were exposed to diethylstilbestrol while in utero have an increased risk of anomalies of the genital tract.

5. Cigarette smoking at the time of conception has been shown to increase the risk of ectopic pregnancy.

6. Assisted reproduction. Several studies have shown that several forms of assisted reproduction have been associated with increased risk of ectopic pregnancies. However, further studies seem to indicate that this risk is associated with concurrent tubal disease.

7. Hormonal imbalance. Excessive levels of estrogen or progesterone may interfere with the normal contractility of the fallopian tube.

8. Previous tubal sterilization. In women who become pregnant after a tubal ligation there is a 16%–50% rate of ectopic pregnancy.

HOW DO WOMEN WITH ECTOPIC PREGNANCY PRESENT?

Typically women who have ectopic pregnancies present with complaints of lower abdominal pain. In addition, they may notice absence of menses, irregular bleeding, or spotting. Most important, these symptoms are present in the setting of a positive pregnancy test. The most common misdiagnoses for ectopic pregnancy include gastrointestinal disorders, normal pregnancy with an ovarian cyst, and pelvic inflammatory disease.

The greatest risk related to an ectopic pregnancy is rupture. As the pregnancy grows outside of the uterus, the embryo begins to enlarge beyond the size of the tube. In combination with the increased blood flow to a growing embryo, the risk of rupturing through the tube means that a woman can lose a significant amount of blood in a very short period of time. Women who have a ruptured ectopic pregnancy classically present with sudden onset of severe lower abdominal pain, possible fainting episode, lightheadedness or dizziness, and a history of irregular bleeding.

HOW IS IT DIAGNOSED?

Initially when a woman presents to her doctor with the complaints described above, a urine pregnancy test is performed. At the same time a blood sample is drawn and sent for the beta human chorionic gonadotropin (B-HCG) level. The B-HCG is the blood test to determine whether a woman is pregnant or not. While a urine pregnancy test can tell whether a woman is pregnant or not, the blood test will give a numeric value that correlates with how far along in the pregnancy a woman is. In normal pregnancies the B-HCG level doubles about every two days. However, in an ectopic pregnancy the rise is less than normal. In addition, the B-HCG level will correlate with certain ultrasound findings. After the initial urine pregnancy test is positive and the blood B-HCG is sent to the lab, an ultrasound is performed. Based on the date of the last menstrual period, an approximate gestational age is determined. A transvaginal ultrasound can reveal evidence of an intrauterine pregnancy as early as five weeks. Since the majority of ectopic pregnancies cannot be seen on ultrasound, we use the presence of an intrauterine pregnancy on ultrasound to rule out an ectopic pregnancy. In addition, if the B-HCG level returns >1,500, we should be able to see evidence of an intrauterine pregnancy on transvaginal ultrasound. If the blood B-HCG level does not correlate with the ultrasound findings, suspicion for an ectopic is raised. If the B-HCG level is too low to reveal an intrauterine pregnancy, the physician is faced with a dilemma and assesses the severity of the patient's current symptoms. If the patient is stable (meaning normal blood pressure and heart rate, able to sit up without getting lightheaded, and having only mild pain), she may be sent home and followed up with another blood B-HCG level. If this second level is double the initial level, then a normal pregnancy is suspected and the ultrasound is repeated. If the level is less than double, then suspicion of an ectopic pregnancy is high.

If the B-HCG rise is abnormal (less than double), then either an ectopic pregnancy or an abnormal intrauterine pregnancy exists. A dilation and currettage performed now can document whether there was abnormal embryonic tissue within the uterus. If it is present, then there was an abnormal intrauterine pregnancy. However, if there is no evidence of embryonic tissue, then an ectopic pregnancy is suspected.

Laparoscopy (the visualization of the pelvic organs using a telescope-like instrument inserted through the belly button) or laparotomy (making an incision and looking directly at the internal organs) is the procedure of choice for the definitive diagnosis of an ectopic pregnancy. In patients who are felt to be unstable, one of these procedures should be undertaken immediately.

Other procedures and tests have been used for the diagnosis of ectopic pregnancy. A serum progesterone level is low in abnormal pregnancies, but the level cannot differentiate between an ectopic and an abnormal pregnancy. Culdocentesis is a procedure where fluid is removed from the abdominal cavity by inserting a needle through the vaginal wall next to the cervix. The fluid removed can help diagnose a ruptured ectopic.

WHAT IS THE TREATMENT?

Once an ectopic pregnancy has been diagnosed, there are two major treatment options based on the severity of the case as well as expectant management.

The majority of cases, including those ruptured, are managed surgically. Laparoscopy or laparotomy is performed, and the ectopic pregnancy is removed. This is done by opening the tube with a small incision and removing the embryo or, if there is significant bleeding or the embryo cannot be fully removed, a portion of the tube is removed.

In a small proportion of the cases it is possible to treat ectopic pregnancies medically with methotrexate. This drug interferes with synthesis of DNA (the building block of chromosomes, which tell cells what to do). The criteria for medical management with methotrexate are that the patient is stable, the tubal pregnancy is unruptured, the size <3.5 cm, and the peak B-HCG is <15,000. Expectant management is undertaken in women who present early, have decreasing B-HCG levels, and are stable. These women must be followed up closely to assure that the levels continue to decline and that they do not develop evidence of rupture. There have been patients whose levels have returned to almost normal and then ruptured, indicating the importance of close monitoring.

WHAT IS THE PROGNOSIS FOR FUTURE PREGNANCY?

Overall, the subsequent conception rate leading to a live birth is about 35%. This number is significantly higher in women who have a history of an unruptured ectopic pregnancy. Thus early diagnosis is extremely important. Women who have had an ectopic pregnancy should tell their physician and be followed closely to assure proper implantation of the embryo.

Premature Rupture of the Fetal Membranes

Kunle Odunsi, MD, PhD, and Paolo Rinaudo, MD

Premature rupture of membranes (PROM) constitutes one of the most important dilemmas in current obstetric practice. The term is applied to leakage of amniotic fluid in the absence of labor, irrespective of gestational age. PROM before 37 weeks' gestation is referred to as preterm premature rupture of membranes (PPROM). Overall, about 10% of all gestations are complicated by PROM. At term, the incidence of PROM varies from 6% to 19%. Nearly all women with PPROM will eventually deliver before term, and the majority will deliver within one week of rupture, regardless of gestational age at the time of membrane rupture.

MECHANISMS OF PROM

The chorioamniotic membranes possess elastic properties. However, there is evidence to suggest that when the membranes are stressed, either by internal pressure due to labor or by infection, they are weakened and have an increased susceptibility to premature rupture.[3] Several studies have shown that both the cell organization of the amniotic membrane and the quality and quantity of membrane collagen are altered in the patient with PROM. Specifically, it appears that type 3 collagen may be reduced in patients with PROM.[4] Additionally, enhanced collagen-destroying activity has been found in prematurely ruptured amniotic membranes.

There is now compelling evidence that infection is a major etiologic factor in a significant proportion of preterm labor and preterm premature rupture of fetal membranes. The most commonly associated organisms found were those causing bacterial vaginosis: *Trichomonas vaginalis*, mycoplasmas, *Chlamydia trachomitis*, *Neisseria gonorrhoeae*, and group B streptococci. In addition, *Bacteroides fragilis*, peptostreptococci, and fusobacteria—bacteria commonly isolated from the amniotic fluid in the presence of preterm labor—and other common vaginal bacteria, including lactobacilli and *Staphylococcus epidermidis*, may release inflammatory mediators that may cause uterine contractions. This leads to cervical change, separation of the chorion from the amnion, and PROM.

Maternal and fetal stress may also cause the release of stress mediators via the hypothalamic-pituitary-adrenal axis, leading to enhanced production of placental corticotrophin-releasing hormone. The latter enhances the release of enzymes and compounds that may lead to PPROM.

Other risk factors for PROM include cigarette smoking,[5] vaginal bleeding, incompetent cervix, and poor nutritional status. Other factors, called not remediable factors, include PROM in a previous pregnancy (recurrence rate of 21%), Ehlers-Danlos syndrome, placenta previa, placental abruption, marginal insertion of the umbilical cord, battledore placenta, multiple gestation, and polyhydramnios.

COMPLICATIONS OF PROM

The consequences of PROM for the neonate fall into three major overlapping categories. The first is the significant neonatal morbidity and mortality associated with prematurity. Second are the complications during labor and delivery that increase the risk for neonatal resuscitation. Third is infection. The morbidity and mortality associated with PROM increase with decreasing gestational age. Maternal complications include infection and increased risk of cesarean section.

Once membranes rupture, the duration of the latency period varies inversely with the gestational age. When PROM occurs between 28 and 34 weeks, 50% are in labor within 24 hours, and 80% to 90% within a week.[6] Maternal infection is termed chorioamnionitis; fetal infection may occur as septicemia, pneumonia, urinary tract infection, or local infections such as omphalitis (infection of the umbilical cord) or conjunctivitis. The incidence of chorioamnionitis in association with PROM varies with the population studied. In prolonged rupture of membranes, the incidence is 3%–15%; it appears to be more common in PPROM, with a frequency of 15% to 25%.[7] Major neonatal infections occur in about 5% of all cases of PPROM, and in 15%–20% of those with chorioamnionitis.

The relative contributions of prematurity and perinatal infections to perinatal mortality are responsible for most of the controversy surrounding the optimal management of PPROM. In most cases, perinatal mortality consequent upon PPROM arises from complications of prematurity such as respiratory distress syndrome, intraventricular hemorrhage, and necrotizing enterocolitis. Thus, in a 26-week gestation, the relative contribution of prematurity to the risks of perinatal morbidity and mortality far outweighs any risks from infection, and all efforts at prolonging pregnancy would seem reasonable. However, in a fetus at 34 weeks, at which point perinatal mortality is not substantially different from that for the fetus at term, the relative contribution of infection becomes more important.

Umbilical cord prolapse occurs more frequently in PROM, with a reported incidence of 1.5%.[8] It has now become clear that cord compression, even without prolapse, is more common in PROM because of the accompanying oligohydramnios.[9] Studies of antepartum testing in patients with PPROM suggest a high incidence of antepartum fetal distress requiring intervention for fetal heart rate patterns consistent with umbilical cord compression occurring even prior to the onset of labor.[10] Vintzileos et al.[11] reported a good correlation between the severity of oligohydramnios and the frequency of severe variable decelerations, low Apgar scores, and perinatal mortality.

The final major complication that may result from PPROM is the fetal deformation syndrome. PROM occurring very early in pregnancy can result in growth retardation, compression anomalies of the fetal face and limbs, and, most important, pulmonary hypoplasia. Sustained adequate amniotic fluid and normal fetal breathing movements are necessary for normal lung growth. Itoh and Itoh[12] reported that fetuses with renal agenesis (insult before four to six weeks) have defects in all three stages of lung development, whereas fetuses with early oligohydramnios (insult before 20 weeks) exhibit nearly normal bronchial branching and cartilage development but have histologically immature alveoli.

Fetal pulmonary hypoplasia has a 90% mortality rate. The reported incidence in PPROM varies between 3%[13] and 28%.[14] Prenatal diagnosis of pulmonary hypoplasia is difficult, and there have been unsuccessful attempts to correlate features such as fetal thoracic dimension, fetal lung length, and absent fetal breathing movements with diagnosis.[15]

MAKING THE DIAGNOSIS OF PROM

The diagnosis of rupture of membranes is based on the logical sequence of history, physical examination, and laboratory testing. In many instances, it is clear from a history of sudden gush of fluid from the vagina and its continuing intermittent trickle. However, most fluid might have escaped and fluid may not be present in the vagina, making it difficult to confirm or refute the diagnosis. Furthermore, fluid may be contaminated with urine, cervical mucus, bathwater, vaginal discharge, blood, or meconium. Because of these difficulties, even when fluid is available, differentiation between amniotic fluid and urine or vaginal secretions is essential. Keirse et al.[16] found that 20% of women with preterm gestations who came to a labor and delivery unit with a primary complaint of "aqueous discharge" did not have ruptured membranes. No one test has been found to be completely accurate, and diagnosis still requires an integration of the clinical history, physical examination, and laboratory testing. Three tests are currently used for diagnosis of PROM: ferning, nitrazine test, and observation of a pool of fluid in the vagina.

Arborization or "fernlike" patterns occur in a variety of body fluids when they are put on a glass slide and allowed to dry, because of the presence of proteins and electrolytes. Positive "ferning" is considered a sign of ruptured membranes. The nitrazine test is probably the most widely used for helping establish the diagnosis of ruptured membranes. Nitrazine is an indicator paper with a narrow set point of pH 6.4–6.8 where it undergoes the characteristic color change to blue in the presence of amniotic fluid. Overall, the combination of history, physical examination, nitrazine testing, and microscopy for ferning should lead to the correct diagnosis of up to 90% of cases of PROM. The question of whether or not to perform vaginal examination in patients with PROM is a controversial area of practice. The most widely held opinion is that a visual speculum examination alone is sufficient to provide most of the information required for management.

MANAGEMENT OF PPROM

The major risks to the baby following PPROM are related to the complications of prematurity. The neonatologist and obstetrician should work as a team to ensure that optimal care is provided for the mother and the fetus. Several studies have shown that small changes in gestational age have significant impact on survival, especially for neonates delivered between 24 and 26 weeks. Morbidity is also dependent on weight and decreases with increasing birth weight.

Since the goal of management in PPROM is prolongation of pregnancy, the most commonly accepted management scheme for the patient at less than 36 weeks is expectant management in the hospital. This consists of careful observation for signs of infection, labor, or fetal distress in an effort to gain time for fetal growth and maturation. Although most patients commit themselves to delivery by going into labor, some do reach term and the timing of delivery must be decided. When the patient reaches 36 or 37 weeks, delivery may be accomplished, but documented lung maturity may permit a somewhat earlier delivery. This expectant approach is complicated by controversies surrounding the efficacy of tocolytic agents to stop uterine contractions, prophylactic antibiotics, corticosteroids to accelerate fetal lung maturation, and amniocentesis for diagnosis of occult infection and fetal lung maturity. In any event, where adequate facilities for intensive perinatal and neonatal care are lacking, it is prudent to refer the patient to a center where such facilities are available.

DOCUMENTATION OF FETAL WELL-BEING IN PROM

PROM is associated with an increased frequency of maternal infection, neonatal infection, and fetal distress during preterm and term labor. The main challenge, therefore, is how to recognize and detect intrauterine infection at its incipient stages. In the United States, analysis of amniotic fluid obtained by amniocentesis is currently the most widely practiced method to determine the presence or absence of bacteria in the amniotic cavity and to determine fetal pulmonary maturity. The most common tests for the detection of bacteria are Gram stain and cultures for aerobic and anaerobic bacteria, including *Mycoplasma* species. In order to improve the efficacy of Gram staining, other markers of infection have been examined, such as amniotic fluid white blood cell count, leukocyte esterase, and glucose. Although there is currently inadequate evidence on the value of amniocentesis in PROM, it would appear that the routine use of transabdominal amniocentesis to detect silent intra-amniotic infection is justified. The amniotic fluid is used to document pulmonary maturity studies. The demonstration of a lecithin:sphingomyelin ratio greater than 2 from the amniocentesis sample or the presence of a phosphatidyl glycerol band in the vaginal pool specimen is usually taken as an indication of pulmonary maturity. Ultrasonography has become an essential part of the evaluation of patients with PPROM. The evaluation includes assessment of dates and size, exclusion of fetal anomalies, and determination of fetal behavior.

ANTIBIOTIC THERAPY IN EXPECTANT MANAGEMENT OF PPROM

The use of prophylactic antibiotics in PPROM can reduce maternal and perinatal risks of infection, and the interval from PROM to delivery may be prolonged (since occult infection is a probable cause of PPROM and preterm labor). In a meta-analysis of antimicrobial therapy in PPROM, Mercer and Arheart[17] showed that antimicrobial treatment offered significant benefit in pregnancy prolongation, and fewer women delivered by twenty-four hours with antimicrobial therapy. There was also a decrease in chorioamnionitis as well as infectious maternal and infant morbidity, including sepsis and pneumonia. However, many questions remain to be answered, including whether or not these findings are applicable to all populations, what is the best antibiotic (including route and duration of therapy), and whether or not a selective approach is feasible, reserving antibiotic therapy for a specific group of patients at higher risk. Until these issues are addressed, the use of antibiotic prophylaxis in PPROM should be individualized, and blanket use should not be regarded as "standard of care" because it may increase iatrogenic morbidity from superinfection due to resistant bacterial species.

CORTICOSTEROIDS AFTER PPROM

The benefit of antenatal corticosteroid therapy has been demonstrated in several randomized controlled trials. The overall reduction in the odds of neonatal respiratory distress syndrome is about 50%.[18] This beneficial effect on respiratory distress syndrome is thought to have a domino effect on other forms of neonatal morbidity, including a 10% and an 80% reduction in the odds of periventricular hemorrhage[19] and necrotizing enterocolitis,[20] respectively. In the light of available evidence, corticosteroid therapy should be initiated as soon as possible in all cases of PPROM from 24 to 34 weeks unless immediate delivery is indicated for chorioamnionitis, antepartum hemorrhage, cord prolapse, or fetal distress. Treatment should consist of dexamethasone by intramuscular injection in two doses at twelve-hour intervals. If the patient remains undelivered after a week, an attempt should be made to assess lung maturity, and the corticosteroid regime repeated if necessary.[21]

TOCOLYSIS IN PPROM

Several prospective randomized controlled trials of tocolytic agents (agents that reduce uterine contractions) in patients with PPROM have been conducted.[22] Overall, there was no difference in pregnancy prolongation beyond twenty-four hours or any difference in any index of perinatal mortality or morbidity measured. Two randomized trials of prophylactic oral tocolytics also failed to show pregnancy prolongation.[23] These data offer no support for suggestions that prophylactic oral tocolysis before the onset of uterine contractions is worthwhile. A possible but unproven advantage of tocolysis lies in the postponement of labor in order to facilitate in utero transfer in PPROM.

PREVIABLE PROM

In cases of PROM very early in pregnancy, survival after delivery at or less than 23 weeks is limited, and neonatal morbidity and mortality after delivery at 24 to 26 weeks are high. If labor or clinical infection is present at initial evaluation of these patients, delivery is indicated. For the remainder of patients, there are two options: expectant management or termination. It is extremely important that the patient be involved in the decision process. Ongoing counseling and psychological support are essential in the management of this morbid pregnancy complication.

MANAGEMENT OF PROM AT TERM

Labor induction or expectant management? The question of whether or not to induce labor immediately when PROM occurs at term is a vexing issue. Immediate induction of labor can lead to higher cesarean section rates (thought to be due to the fact that the cervix was unripe in many cases). However, a careful, large randomized controlled trial which included 5,041 women with PROM at term[24] showed that induction of labor with intravenous oxytocin, induction of labor with vaginal prostaglandin E2 gel, and expectant management are all reasonable options for women and their babies if membranes rupture before the start of labor at term, since they result in similar rates of neonatal infection and cesarean delivery. However, induction of labor with intravenous oxytocin resulted in a lower risk of maternal infection, and women viewed induction of labor more positively than expectant management.

Should prophylactic antibiotics be used? In Centers for Disease Control and Prevention recommendations for preventing early onset neonatal group B streptococcal (GBS) disease, rupture of membrane for more than eighteen hours was classified as a risk factor for GBS infection, and antibiotic chemoprophylaxis with penicillin or ampicillin was recommended. For women who are allergic to penicillin, clindamycin or erythromycin would be a suitable alternative.

SUMMARY

Premature rupture of the fetal membranes is an obstetric enigma, and several aspects of management of PPROM and PROM at term remain controversial. Although clinical judgment, physician experience, and careful individualization of management often come into play, certain principles are widely accepted as being essential. The issues to be addressed by the obstetrician caring for the patient presenting with PROM are: Are the membranes indeed ruptured? What is the gestational age? Should the cervix be examined? Should labor be suppressed? Should labor be induced? Should the mother be transported? Is there any reason not to administer glucocorticoids? How and when should delivery be accomplished? These questions are best answered based on the best available evidence. Future studies are warranted to identify the optimal methods of prolongation of the latency interval while avoiding compression deformities and pulmonary hypoplasia in cases where membrane rupture occurs very early in pregnancy, as well as the optimal mode of surveillance in these pregnancies.[25]

Substance Abuse During Pregnancy

Ashley Wivel, MD

Substance abuse during pregnancy poses a threat to the health and well-being of both the mother and her unborn child. It is difficult to know exactly how many women abuse alcohol and drugs during their pregnancies, but the problem is clearly of concerning size. About 15% of women who present for prenatal care have a positive urine test for one or more of the following: alcohol, marijuana, cocaine, and opiates (such as heroin).

This is worrisome not only because almost every substance of abuse freely crosses the placenta into the fetus but also because of the risky behaviors that can be associated with substance abuse, including unsafe sex, exchanging sex for drugs and money, and engaging in physically unsafe behavior.

Although many of the substances described below may cause fetal death, this article takes a broader look at the effects of both licit and illicit substances on a woman and her fetus. This article summarizes what is known about the effects of certain substances during pregnancy, in the hope that education will help women to understand the risks of using addictive substances during pregnancy and will help them to choose to abstain while they are pregnant.

TOBACCO

Tobacco smoke is a highly complex substance containing many possibly harmful ingredients, including nicotine, tar, carbon monoxide, and cyanide. All of these appear to contribute to the health problems affecting mothers who smoke, including respiratory illnesses, peptic ulcer disease, esophageal reflux, and, in the long term, cancer.

Nicotine is particularly problematic during pregnancy because it tends to make blood vessels constrict, which decreases blood flow to the placenta (which translates into less oxygen and nutrients for the fetus). In addition to decreasing blood flow, smoking can lead to a complication called placental abruption, in which the placenta detaches from the wall of the uterus before the fetus is ready to be born. One in 500 cases of severe abruption leads to fetal death.

In general, smoking is associated with an increased frequency of miscarriage, the risk being increased 1.2-fold for every ten cigarettes smoked per day. A report by the Surgeon General in 1983 estimated that 4,600 infants died each year in the United States as a result of their mother's smoking during pregnancy. Babies of smokers also tend to be born prematurely and to have lower birth weights, with birth weight reduction being directly related to the number of cigarettes smoked each day. Increased rates of neonatal death and of sudden infant death syndrome have also been observed. The long-term effects of smoking are still under investigation, but smoking during pregnancy has been associated with impaired growth after birth, impaired intellectual development, and behavioral disorders including hyperactivity and attention deficit disorders.

ALCOHOL

Alcohol use during pregnancy is a significant problem: it has been estimated that as many as 1 in 300 infants are born with some stigmata of fetal alcohol exposure. The best described stigmata are part of the fetal alcohol syndrome (FAS), which includes (1) prenatal and postnatal growth retardation, (2) central nervous system involvement, and (3) characteristic facial features. The central nervous system effects include tremulousness, poor suckling, abnormal muscle tone, hyperactivity, attention deficit, and mental retardation. The typical facial features include microcephaly (a small head), a thin upper lip, a short, upturned nose, a flattened nasal bridge, and general underdevelopment of the midface area.

Drinking patterns vary among women, and it appears that heavier drinking is associated with more congenital problems. However, no safe level of alcohol intake during pregnancy has ever been defined. Both binge drinking and daily drinking increase the risk of fetal abnormalities, such as FAS, and of fetal death. Alcohol use during pregnancy is associated with an increased incidence of second trimester miscarriage in moderate-to-heavy drinkers. Abruption of the placenta and breech presentation also appear to be more common in fetuses with FAS.

Other fetal defects that may be associated with alcohol exposure include congenital heart defects, brain abnormalities, spinal bifida, limb defects, urinary tract defects, and genital defects.

MARIJUANA

Marijuana is the most commonly used illicit substance in the United States, and it is the most common recreational drug used during pregnancy. It is important to know that the psychoactive ingredient in marijuana, 1,9-tetrahydrocannabinol (THC), accumulates in fat. THC is broken down by the liver before being excreted, but it may stay in fat tissue for days. Thus, the effects of using marijuana may persist for some time. Marijuana has multiple effects on the mother, including producing tachycardia (a fast heart rate), exercise intolerance, bronchitis, sinusitis, and pharyngitis. The effects of marijuana on the fetus are the subject of some debate. There are reports in the literature of decreased body length, intrauterine growth retardation, neurobehavioral effects, and an increased incidence of prematurity. These findings, however, have not been consistent in all studies.

COCAINE

Cocaine is a potent stimulator of the brain that produces the euphoria experienced by the user, and it has been estimated that 10% of the obstetric population uses cocaine. Cocaine's other effects, however, can be quite dangerous. The mother may experience a number of serious side effects, including fast heart rate, dangerously high blood pressure, a heart attack, irregular heartbeat, muscle twitching, seizures, stroke, increased body temperature, and even sudden death. The effects of these conditions on the fetus can be dramatic and may be fatal. Placental abruption is seen in up to 8% of cocaine abusers. Miscarriages during the first trimester are estimated to occur at a rate approaching 40%. Babies of cocaine abusers tend to have low birth weights and intrauterine growth retardation and are more likely to be premature.

Cocaine, like nicotine, tends to constrict blood vessels, sometimes with dire consequences. Constriction of blood vessels is thought to be responsible for certain fetal abnormalities associated with cocaine abuse, including failure to form part of the intestines and failure to form the limbs properly. Congenital heart defects and urinary tract abnormalities have also been observed. The effects on the fetus's central nervous system vary from major disruptive brain anomalies to disordered behaviors seen in newborns. Newborns tend to have depressed interactive behavior and to have difficulty organizing their responses to the outside world. Research is currently under way to study the long-term effects of cocaine use during pregnancy.

OPIATES

Heroin and methadone are the drugs in this class most frequently used during pregnancy. Although neither causes congenital abnormalities, they pose a significant threat not only because use of heroin involves needles, and thus may increase the risk for HIV infection, but also because withdrawal can be fatal to the fetus. Problems the mother may encounter from using heroin include overdose, skin and subcutaneous tissue infections, inflammation of the veins used for injection, endocarditis (infection of the tissues of the heart), and urinary tract infection. And there is an increased incidence of inflammation and infection of the placenta and the uterus. Opiate use is also associated with an increased risk of premature labor and delivery, low birth weight, fetal distress, and neonatal infections.

Withdrawal in the mother can cause agitation, tearing, runny nose, yawning, perspiration, abdominal and uterine cramps, diarrhea, and muscle aches. Withdrawal in the mother may be fatal to the fetus because it results in hyperactivity, hypoxia (lack of oxygen to the fetus), and meconium (passage of the fetus's first bowel movement while still in the uterus, which is a sign that the fetus is in distress). All babies born to mothers using heroin will be addicted to the drug, and 80% of those born to mothers on methadone will be addicted to opiates. The addicted babies will undergo the neonatal withdrawal syndrome. The symptoms begin twelve to twenty four hours after birth and include high-pitched crying, frantic fist sucking, frantic searching for food, and tremulousness. The baby can have seizures, display a disrupted sleep-wake cycle, and have rigid muscles. The long-term effects of maternal opiate use have yet to be defined. In terms of using heroin versus methadone, methadone is thought to be better because the levels of the drug are more constant and there is much less likelihood that the mother will withdraw.

AMPHETAMINES

Amphetamines are central nervous system stimulants with effects on the brain similar to those of cocaine. Tolerance develops with use, leading the user to need more to achieve the same euphoric feelings. Amphetamines may cause the user to be hyperactive, to be paranoid, to hallucinate, to suffer insomnia, and to be malnourished secondary to a decreased appetite. These drugs can be used intravenously, which may increase the risk for HIV infection. Very little is known about what amphetamines do to the fetus. Although no defined set of congenital anomalies exists, there is some indication that amphetamine use may be associated with placental abruption, prematurity, and low birth weight.

HALLUCINOGENS

The most commonly used hallucinogens are lysergic acid diethylamide (LSD, "acid") and phencyclidine (PCP, "angel dust"). The effects on the mother are significant because users tend to put themselves in dangerous situations that can lead to harm of the mother and her fetus. Users can become violent, which may lead to direct trauma. The direct effects of these substances on the fetus are not well defined. There are some reports in the literature suggesting that use of hallucinogens is associated with decreased birth weight and decreased head circumference, but these findings may be attributable to environmental factors. Neonates, nonetheless, can withdraw from hallucinogens with such symptoms as tremors, jitteriness, and irritability. The long-term effects are still being investigated and may involve developmental delays.

CONCLUSIONS

Using drugs and alcohol during pregnancy can cause a variety of problems for both the mother and her fetus, ranging from malnutrition in the mother to major congenital abnormalities in the fetus involving vital structures such as the heart or brain. There are a few points to remember. There is no safe level of use of any of the substances discussed above. Even if a substance of abuse does not have an obvious syndrome of abnormalities associated with it, it may affect the fetus in ways that will not become apparent until the baby has reached school age or adulthood. Also, it is often the environment in which substances are abused and the fact that when one substance is abused, it is more likely that multiple substances will be abused, that pose the greatest threat to the mother and the fetus. And, finally, the time to deal with substance abuse is before pregnancy begins, because many of the vital organs are formed during the first sixty days of pregnancy, before some women are even aware that they are pregnant.

Hypertensive Disorders in Pregnancy

Tanja Pejovic, MD, PhD

Hypertensive disorders are the most common medical complications of pregnancy and the major cause of maternal and infant disease and death worldwide. They comprise two different entities. Pregnancy-induced hypertension (PIH) appears for the first time during pregnancy and is reversed by delivery. Chronic hypertension is a preexisting condition unrelated to but coinciding with pregnancy; it may be unmasked for the first time during pregnancy and does not resolve with delivery.

Regardless of pregnant or nonpregnant state, hypertension is in many cases the result of small vessels' spasm (vasoconstriction). Therefore, the major risks to the fetus result from decreased placental perfusion, leading to decreased supply of oxygen and nutrients necessary for fetal growth and well-being. Maternal risks include hypoperfusion of major organs such as kidneys, liver, and brain. Hypertension may also lead to brain edema and hemorrhage and to seizures.

Management of hypertensive disorders in pregnancy requires very careful maternal observation and measurement of fetal-placental function and fetal maturity, in order to balance maternal risks of continuing pregnancy against risk to the infant of premature extrauterine existence. Even mild hypertension may rapidly lead to catastrophic complications, such as placental abruption or seizures, that have no parallel in nonpregnant individuals with mild hypertension. By timely recognition and treatment of the disease, these complications may be prevented. However, while therapeutic agents are useful, it is essential to understand their pharmacokinetics and recognize possible side effects to both mother and fetus.

CLASSIFICATION

The terminology used to classify hypertensive disorders of pregnancy has been inconsistent and confusing. More than sixty names in English and forty in German have been applied to these conditions. In the past, hypertensive disorders of pregnancy were commonly called toxemia of pregnancy, which reflected the opinion that these disorders resulted from circulating toxins. This is now known not to be true, and the term "toxemia" has been abandoned by the medical community. Therefore, the Committee on Terminology of the American College of Obstetricians and Gynecologists (ACOG)[26] prepared a classification system for hypertension in pregnancy that was approved by the National Institutes of Health in 1990 and is now used all over the world.

Chronic Hypertension

The ACOG Committee on Terminology defines hypertension as blood pressure higher than 140/90. Chronic hypertension is defined as hypertension present before pregnancy or diagnosed before the 20th week of gestation. Hypertension that persists beyond the 42nd day postpartum is also classified as chronic hypertension.

PIH: Preeclampsia and Eclampsia

The definition/diagnosis of preeclampsia includes elevated blood pressure, the abnormal presence of proteins in the urine (proteinuria), and leakage of blood plasma into the tissues (edema). The blood pressure in preeclampsia must either (a) exceed the blood pressure before 20 gestational weeks by 30 mm Hg systolic and 15 mm Hg diastolic or (b) be more than 140/90 after 20 weeks. Since it is sometimes difficult to define elevated blood pressure (e.g., when systolic pressure is elevated but diastolic is normal), Page and Christianson[27] advocated the use of mean arterial pressure (MAP) as a criterion for elevated blood pressure in pregnancy: MAP= (syst BP+ [2 × diastol BP])/3. Proteinuria is defined as excretion of 0.1g/l of proteins in a randomly sampled urine specimen or 0.3g/l in a twenty-four-hour specimen. Edema is diagnosed by tissue swelling and/or increase in body weight due to water retention.

Preeclampsia may be classified as mild or severe. One or more of the following may indicate severe preeclampsia:

1. The blood pressure is > 160 systolic or > 110 diastolic, registered on at least two occasions at least six hours apart in a patient on bed rest
2. Proteinuria is > 5g/24 hours
3. Urine production is < 400 ml/24h (oliguria)
4. Cerebral/visual disturbances
5. Epigastric pain
6. Pulmonary edema, cyanosis
7. Impaired liver function
8. Thrombocytopenia.

Criteria for mild preeclampsia include the following, documented on two occasions, four hours apart:

1. Blood pressure of 140/90 or MAP>105
2. Proteinuria > 0.3g/l in twenty-four-hour urine sample.

Eclampsia is preeclampsia accompanied by seizures. It has been known since Hippocrates' time as a convulsive disease occurring in pregnant women, but was not distinguished from epilepsy until the nineteenth century. However, the path from preeclampsia to eclampsia is highly variable. In some cases the preeclampsia is very mild, and seizures can occur even in a patient with only elevated blood pressure or without proteinuria.

Transient hypertension is an elevated blood pressure after 20 weeks of pregnancy or in the first twenty-four hours postpartum that is not associated with other signs of preeclampsia or chronic hypertension, and that disappears ten days after delivery.

PREECLAMPSIA SUPERIMPOSED UPON CHRONIC HYPERTENSION

This diagnosis is made in a pregnant patient with known hypertension when the baseline blood pressure increases by 30 mm Hg systolic and 15 mm Hg diastolic, or 20 mm Hg MAP, together with edema and proteinuria.

PATHOPHYSIOLOGY OF PREECLAMPSIA-ECLAMPSIA

The major pathophysiologic feature of preeclampsia-eclampsia is vasospasm. This concept, first introduced 1918 by Franz Volhard, is based upon direct observation of small vessels in the retina, nail beds, and bulbar conjunctiva, and histologic examination of various organs during preeclampsia. Vasospasm causes increased resistance to blood flow, leading to arterial hypertension and damage to the endothelium of blood vessels. The areas of damaged endothelium become sites of platelet and fibrinogen deposition and thrombus formation, which, together with hypoxia caused by vasospasm, weaken the vessel wall and lead to hemorrhage, necrosis, and organ dysfunction.

One of the explanations for the generalized vasospasm in preeclampsia is increased vascular responsivity to normal concentrations of endogenous pressors (angiotensin II, norepinephrine, vasopressin).[28] Similarly, women with chronic hypertension who are refractory to angiotensin II between 21 and 25 gestational weeks start to lose this refractoriness after 27 weeks.[29] The blunted response to angiotensin II in normal pregnancy is probably caused by endothelial synthesis of prostaglandins.[30] Prostacyclin, one of the prostaglandins, is a very potent vasodilator produced by the endothelium. Vessels of preeclamptic women and umbilical veins of their fetuses produce far less prostacyclin compared with normal pregnancy.[31] Nitric oxide is another vasodilator produced by endothelium that acts synergistically with prostacyclin.[32] Nitric oxide production is also decreased because of endothelial cell injury. Therefore it seems clear that endothelial injury and decreased production of vasodilators play a major role in pathogenesis of pregnancy-induced hypertension.

MATERNAL AND FETAL CONSEQUENCES OF PREECLAMPSIA-ECLAMPSIA

Deterioration of maternal organs secondary to vasospasm and hypoperfusion is a direct consequence of PIH. Similarly, deterioration of fetal status is caused by vasoconstriction and placental hypoperfusion.

CARDIOVASCULAR SYSTEM

Blood pressure elevation in severe PIH constitutes an acute threat to the mother. Pressures as high as 200/120 are sometimes encountered. Cerebral hemorrhage and cardiac decompensation are potential complications of such blood pressure increases, and heart failure is one of the most common causes of maternal death due to preeclampsia; it is rarely encountered in young women who are otherwise healthy. Circulatory collapse (sudden decrease in systolic blood pressure to less than 70 mm Hg) may occur a few hours after delivery. Another serious complication is pulmonary edema as a part of generalized edema. However, pulmonary edema is far more frequently a consequence of treatment and not of PIH itself; typical causes of iatrogenic fluid overload are aggressive replacement of fluids after cesarean section and prolonged administration of oxytocin.

CEREBRAL INVOLVEMENT

Vascular resistance in cerebral vessels is unaltered in normal pregnancy, but is increased in 50% of women with PIH. In some patients this leads to cerebral hemorrhage, one of the common causes of death in women with PIH. Some patients with severe preeclampsia may have cerebral edema, which occurs by the same mechanisms as generalized or pulmonary edema. Headache, altered consciousness, and blurred vision are common symptoms of cerebral edema. They also typically precede eclamptic seizures.

LIVER FUNCTION

Liver involvement is seen in about 10% of women with severe preeclampsia: a variety of liver functions may be deranged.[33] Most commonly, transaminases are mildly elevated, as are bilirubin levels. Liver functions usually return to normal once preeclampsia is treated by delivery of the fetus.

RENAL FUNCTION

Glomerular filtration rate increases in normal pregnancy, and therefore the serum concentrations of creatinine, urea, and uric acid decrease. In preeclampsia, vasospasm and glomerular endothelial swelling lead to a reduction of glomerular filtration rate of 25% below that of normal pregnancy. Serum creatinine is rarely elevated in preeclampsia, but uric acid is commonly increased. In some studies, uric acid levels of more than 5 mg/dl have been associated with poor fetal outcome.[34]

HEMATOLOGICAL CHANGES

Most prominent hematological changes involve plasma volume and hematocrit, clotting factors, and platelets. In severe preeclampsia there is a reduction in plasma volume that may be indicated by rise in hematocrit. In 20% of patients with severe preeclampsia there is evidence of increased consumption of coagulation factors.[35] The best indicators of the activation of the clotting system are decreased concentrations of plasma antithrombin III (a substance that inhibits coagulation by preventing reaction between thrombin and fibrinogen) and a decrease in the ratio of clotting factor VIII activity to factor VIII antigen. Low platelet count (< 150,000/mm) is also a common finding in preeclamptic patients. Repeated platelet-count testing is an important aid in the management of established hypertensive disease in pregnancy.

THE HELLP SYNDROME

There is a syndrome of hemolysis, elevated liver enzymes, and low platelets (HELLP) in severe preeclampsia.[36] Criteria for the diagnosis of this syndrome include (1) hemolysis, defined by abnormal peripheral blood smear and increased bilirubin (>1.2 mg/dl); (2) elevated liver enzymes, defined as increased alanine liver transferase (ALT > 70 u/l) and increased lactate dehydrogenase (LDH > 600 u/l); and a platelet count less than 100,000/ml. Not all women have all of these findings. It is essential to understand that this syndrome may develop even in women with mild preeclampsia (i.e., with no severe hypertension).[37] Patients may present with the syndrome either before delivery or shortly thereafter. Usually patients present before term, complaining of malaise, epigastric pain or pain under the right diaphragm, nausea and vomiting, and some symptoms similar to those of viral infection; they are often misdiagnosed as having some other medical condition. Pregnancies complicated by HELLP syndrome are associated with poor maternal and fetal outcome. Most HELLP patients require blood product transfusions and are at increased risk of developing acute renal failure, pulmonary edema, pleural effusions, and hepatic rupture. Moreover, these patients are at increased risk for placental abruption and disseminated intravascular coagulopathy.

During the course of the disease it is essential to establish fetal well-being by continuous fetal heart monitoring and ultrasound examinations. In the postpartum period, the majority of patients with HELLP syndrome manifest symptoms within forty-eight hours. Eighty percent of these patients were diagnosed with preeclampsia prior to delivery, while 20% had no such evidence before delivery or intrapartum. Patients with this syndrome should be treated at specialized obstetrical care centers. The first priority is to assess and stabilize the maternal condition, particularly to control bleeding and coagulation abnormalities. The next step is to evaluate fetal well-being, using fetal heart monitoring and ultrasound examination. Then a decision must be made whether immediate delivery is indicated. Amniocentesis may be recommended in patients at less than 34 weeks of gestation, but must be balanced against risks of bleeding complications. The presence of this syndrome is NOT an indication for cesarean delivery, which may be detrimental to both mother and the fetus. Patients with delayed resolution of HELLP syndrome after delivery are typically treated with fresh frozen plasma transfusions.

PLACENTA

In pregnancies complicated by preeclampsia there is an inadequate maternal response to placentation (i.e., a fraction of spiral uterine arterioles fail to dilate in the same way as in normal pregnancy, thus decreasing the blood supply to the fetus.[38] Electron microscopic studies have shown characteristic damage to endothelial cells somewhat similar to that of vessels in transplanted but rejected kidneys. This observation has led to the suggestion that immunological mechanisms (i.e., rejection of the fetus by the maternal immune system) may be operative in preeclampsia.[39]

MANAGEMENT OF PREECLAMPSIA

Delivery is the only cure for preeclampsia. The ultimate goal of treatment is always maternal safety first, then the delivery of a live, mature newborn. Beyond hospitalization for preeclampsia and the monitoring of blood pressure, biochemical tests, and fetal well-being, the major goal is prevention of eclampsia. The majority of eclamptic episodes occur in labor or the early postpartum period. The agent of choice for seizure prevention is magnesium sulfate, which typically prevents seizures without sedating the mother. Magnesium sulfate is given intravenously. Normal magnesium concentration in serum is 1.8–2.0mEq/l; therapeutic concentrations for anticonvulsive purposes are 4–7mEq/l. At magnesium levels above 7mEq/l, signs of toxicity appear (loss of patellar reflex). Excessive accumulation of magnesium can be fatal: respiratory depression/arrest occurs at levels of 10–15mEq/l, and cardiac arrest ensues when magnesium concentration reaches 30mEq/l. The major advantage of magnesium sulfate is that it is very safe for the fetus and neonate.[40]

Although at present there is no proven method to prevent preeclampsia, several studies have indicated a beneficial effect of low-dose (60–80mg) aspirin prophylaxis to prevent growth retardation.[41] Aspirin reduces generation of platelet-derived vasoconstrictors and thus alleviates the basic pathologic changes in PIH. However, the long-term effects of aspirin-induced inhibition of prostaglandin synthesis on fetal homeostasis are not known, and this type of therapy is reserved for women at high risk for development of preeclampsia.

Antihypertensive agents are not routinely given to women with preeclampsia because there is no evidence that it improves fetal well-being or risk of seizures in the mother. Therapy is reserved for women with severe hypertension (blood pressures more than 160/110), to decrease risks of intracranial bleeding. Ideally, blood pressure should be lowered to mildly elevated levels to keep good placental perfusion. Alpha-methyldopa (Aldomet) is the preferred agent.

Labor is usually uneventful in preeclamptic women. Pain control by epidural anesthesia may be provided. The feared complications of this type of anesthesia are sympathetic blockade, pooling of blood, and hypotension with compromise of placental perfusion and fetal stress.

PROGNOSES

The perinatal mortality rate is higher for infants of preeclamptic women.[42] Causes of infant death are placental insufficiency and placental abruption, leading to intrauterine death or prematurity.[43] The perinatal mortality rate is highest in preeclampsia superimposed on preexisting hypertensive disease. Growth restriction is also very common in infants of preeclamptic mothers and increases in severity with increasing maternal blood pressure.[44] However, careful observation of intrauterine well-being has decreased the perinatal infant mortality rate in recent years.

Preeclampsia usually resolves promptly and completely after delivery. Proteinuria resolves within one week, and hypertension within two weeks. The risk of recurrent preeclampsia in subsequent pregnancies is 10%–25% if the disease is diagnosed in the third trimester and as high as 60%–70% if the disease is diagnosed in the second trimester.

Loss and Multifetal Pregnancies

David Jones, MD

Women with multifetal pregnancies (twins, triplets, and more) face pregnancy loss just as women with singletons do; however, they also face issues involving losses in which certain aspects are unique to their multiple gestations. In the simplest case, women with twins suffer fetal losses through the "vanishing twin syndrome." The advent of widespread ultrasound use has shown that many twin pregnancies suffer the loss of one twin quite early, and were ultrasound not available, neither the patient nor the caregiver would have recognized the pregnancy as anything but a singleton pregnancy. Sebire et al. evaluated pregnancies at 10–14 weeks with transvaginal ultrasound and determined that about 5% of all twin pregnancies have a demise of one (3.5%) or both (1.5%) twins at that time.[45] Obviously, unrecognized losses do not cause families to suffer loss. In cases where the losses are recognized, feelings of loss often seem muted compared to cases of loss of a singleton. The reason for the milder reaction may be due to a feeling that the pregnancy hasn't miscarried and there is still a viable fetus, due to ambivalent feelings about having twins, or simply due to the fact that these losses are very early and in many cases a fetus (or even fetal heartbeat) was never seen, so the sense of bonding was less.

Beyond the case of the vanishing twin, women with multiple gestations may be faced with three other broad categories of fetal loss with special implications: the elective reduction of a high order (arguably triplets or more) pregnancy to a low order one to improve outcome for the fetuses, the potential loss of a normal fetus when the selective termination of an abnormal twin is performed, and the issues of fetal and neonatal loss surrounding preterm interventions when one twin is severely compromised in utero and the other is healthy.

In general, twins deliver earlier than singletons, triplets earlier than twins; the more fetuses in the womb, the earlier the average delivery. Likewise, while many preterm and extremely preterm infants survive, the earlier one delivers, the higher the risk of serious and possibly lifelong complications. In recent years, the increased use of assisted reproduction technologies has resulted in a rise in the number of triplets and higher-order multiple gestations. While it is clear that this has been a godsend to many couples with long histories of infertility, it has also placed many in the uncomfortable circumstance of carrying triplets and quadruplets with a high potential for one, two, or more children to be born with major, lifelong handicaps including lung disease, mental retardation, seizure disorders, blindness, and cerebral palsy. Consequently, as early as 1986, physicians were reporting on reductions of high order pregnancies to low order ones. This procedure has been refined and has become more widely available. Studies have been fairly convincing that quadruplet pregnancies which are reduced do better than those that are not. While the data for triplets are not as clear, early evidence suggests there is some improvement in outcomes. It does not appear that triplets reduced to twins do quite as well as natural twins, however.

Couples now are routinely informed of this procedure and face two obvious issues. First, they have been trying very hard to get pregnant and have gone to the extremes of high-tech interventions, only to be faced with a decision on whether to terminate one of their much-desired fetuses in order to improve the chances for the others. Many women who choose to undergo reduction experience feelings of loss. Berkowitz et al. found that 65% of women had acute feelings of emotional pain and stress, 70% mourned for their lost fetuses, and 37% had an anniversary grief reaction.[46] Although persistent depressive symptoms were mild, nearly 18% experienced lingering guilt or sadness and anger. Despite these feelings, 93% of the women said they would make the choice to undergo reduction again. A second consideration is that the procedure carries a risk of causing a miscarriage of the whole pregnancy. Fortunately, this complication is uncommon in experienced hands. In a recent series of 400 patients undergoing reductions, 92% delivered one or more infants after 24 weeks' gestation. The risk of miscarriage was 7.3% in triplets, 8.4% in quadruplets, 6.1% in quintuplets, and 17.6% in those with six or more fetuses. Nonetheless, when a miscarriage occurs, the reactions of grief and anger may be significant, given that the patient's decision to undergo reduction has led to the loss of a much-desired and worked-for pregnancy.

A similarly complicated decision faces parents with multiple gestations in which one fetus has an abnormality and the other(s) is(are) normal. While women carrying singleton pregnancies may face the decision to terminate an abnormal pregnancy, women with twins must consider the possibility that their decision could affect the normal fetus. It has been shown that the selective termination of the abnormal fetus is associated with a 3%–8% risk of miscarriage. The emotional strain on a couple brought about by the discovery of a fetal abnormality is complicated by the finding that selective termination of the nonpresenting twin (the one farther from the cervix) lowers the risk of preterm delivery compared to the risk for twins. Should the couple terminate to improve the chances for the normal one? What if they miscarry and lose both? What if they choose not to terminate and the abnormal twin induces a complication that results in a preterm delivery with damage to or loss of the healthy one? No matter what decision they make, they may look back on it with regret if they suffer a loss of both children— on top of the feeling of loss.

Finally, parents of twins may face circumstances in which complications result in the compromise of one twin, and decisions must be made on how to manage the pregnancy. As with all of our previously listed circumstances, patients are called upon to make decisions that may result in the death or compromise of a normal fetus, making the emotions relating to the loss more difficult compared to the case when extraneous factors bring about the loss. There are two subsets of this situation: the case of identical twins with a shared placenta, and the case of nonidentical twins or identical twins with separate placentas. It is sometimes hard to distinguish between the two during pregnancy, particularly if a patient's first visit is relatively late in gestation. In the first case, a situation arises in which one twin becomes severely compromised, such as when an abnormal placenta leads to poor feeding and oxygenation. The compromised fetus can be "starved" to the point of damage and, ultimately, death. Cesarean delivery may be the only option offered to improve the outcome for that fetus; however, delivery of both twins would be performed. Depending on gestational age, this could expose the healthy twin to the complications of prematurity. Parents may be faced with a decision to risk the life of the healthy twin in an attempt to save the sick one, or to sacrifice the sick twin so as not to expose the healthy twin to unnecessary risks.

In the subset of cases with identical twins having a shared placenta, it can be more complicated. Investigators have reported numerous cases of identical twin pregnancies (with shared placentas) in which the demise of one twin caused damage to the other. While the early hypothesis was that something was released from the dead fetus which damaged the other one, more recently it has been hypothesized that the loss of blood pressure in the dead twin results in the live twin pumping blood across to the other one, with a transient loss in blood pressure causing the damage. Unfortunately, studies have not clearly established the level of concern we should have. Estimates of the risk of major morbidity or mortality to the surviving fetus range from very low to 46%. In one report, while there were no cases of damage to the surviving fetus, a high incidence of fetal distress was noted among women retaining a living fetus in utero for a week or more. A final consideration is that the markers for damage don't appear until weeks after the damage has occurred. Unless an impending demise is expected and occurs while a patient is being monitored, there is no way to know whether the healthy fetus suffered a hypotensive crisis, which should produce changes in the fetal heart rate. Thus, parents are sometimes asked to be involved in making decisions with limited data to guide them.

As when considering the issues surrounding loss in the multiple pregnancy, one other factor separates this pregnancy from the singleton pregnancy. When couples suffer a fetal demise in a singleton pregnancy, they either miscarry or undergo a procedure to end the pregnancy. Few mothers desire to carry the dead fetus for more than a few days, and most desire to end the pregnancy quickly. In the case of the multiple gestation with one demise, the mother is often called upon to continue carrying the dead fetus for weeks or months. This may have implications for her grieving process as well as for her feelings toward the surviving twin. Caregivers must recognize that the subsequent birth of a healthy baby will be a time of sorrow as well as joy. We must be careful not to adopt the attitude of "don't complain, be grateful—at least you got one healthy baby." We must take the time to acknowledge and affirm the appropriateness of the couple's emotions of loss while letting them see that they have much to be thankful for.

Thus, the issues surrounding the losses incurred in multiple gestations are frequently more complicated than losses in the singleton, but the emotions are the same. The primary difference is that in many cases, parents are forced to make decisions which have a direct impact on, and sometimes bring about damage or death to, one or more of the fetuses. This may alter the normal feelings of pain, stress, and anger that occur when fetal losses are completely outside the control of the parents.

Infection and Pregnancy Loss

Jacob Tangir, MD

Infectious agents have long been recognized as a cause of spontaneous abortion and perinatal mortality (the perinatal period is from the 22nd week of pregnancy to the 28th day after birth). Scientific understanding of this phenomenon has helped in developing effective preventive measures and treatment for many of these infections. It is important for pregnant women to know the basic mechanism of infections that can potentially affect pregnancy outcome, and how to prevent such infections.

In general there are three major mechanisms by which an infectious agent can affect pregnancy outcome: ascending infections, transplacental infection, and infections acquired through the birth canal. Ascending infections occur when microorganisms residing in the external genitalia of the pregnant women gain access to the amniotic sac. This can debilitate the sac and eventually rupture it. The infectious agent then spreads over the amniotic fluid. At this point the fetus can become infected by aspirating the microorganisms to the lungs, by swallowing them, or by penetration to the ear canal. Also, the inflammatory reaction on the amniotic sac triggered by the infection could initiate labor. In cases of transplacental infection the mother must have the infection along with the presence of circulating microorganisms in the blood. They penetrate the placenta and affect its functioning and also can invade the fetus. Some microorganisms cannot ascend to the amniotic sac nor cross the placental barrier. They colonize the female external genital tract. During the delivery the fetus becomes contaminated by exposure to maternal blood and secretions in the birth canal.

Less common routes of neonatal infection include breast milk and infections acquired in the neonatal intensive care unit or nursery. In terms of the timing, any microorganism that seriously affects the fetus or the mother in the first 20 weeks of pregnancy can cause fetal death and subsequent spontaneous abortion. If the infection occurs between 20 and 37 weeks, it can cause preterm labor and delivery. Preterm delivery is associated with low birth weight and with increased complications as well as neonatal mortality. Finally, infants that acquire infections during passage through the birth canal can develop neonatal infections, which in some cases spread to produce sepsis and death during the first days of life. Following is a brief review of common infections that can complicate pregnancy outcome. Preventive measures and treatment will be discussed when appropriate.

SYPHILIS

Syphilis is a sexually transmitted disease caused by the microorganism *Treponema pallidum*. The incidence of syphilis had been declining since the 1950s and the introduction of penicillin therapy. However, there was an increase in its incidence in the United States that peaked in 1990 and has slowly decreased since then. Many investigators have reported a strong association of maternal syphilis with drug abuse, lack of prenatal care, and race.

The syphilis infectious agent readily crosses the placenta and infects the fetus, causing congenital syphilis. Usually multiple fetal internal organs are affected (e.g., lungs, liver, spleen, and pancreas). The frequency of congenital syphilis varies, depending on the duration and stage of the maternal infection. Fetuses born to mothers with recent infection (primary or secondary) are more likely to be infected than those of mothers with latent disease. The complications of untreated syphilis are well described in reports from the preantibiotic era. Approximately two-thirds of the cases are complicated by perinatal death, preterm labor, or intrauterine growth retardation. Approximately 40% to 50% of the neonates have symptomatic congenital syphilis with a variety of symptoms and damages. More recently, an observational study from a large medical center serving an inner-city population showed a rate of 18.4 cases of congenital syphilis per 10,000 births. Of these, 34% were stillborn, and preterm labor was significantly more common than in nonaffected pregnancies. The resultant perinatal mortality rate in that series was 464 per 1,000. Fortunately, syphilis is relatively easy to diagnose and to treat if there is adequate prenatal care. Usually the diagnosis is made by demonstrating specific antibodies in serologic testing (obtained from blood sampling). The most common test is called VDRL. Because of the devastating effects of congenital syphilis and the effectiveness of the treatment, every pregnant woman should have a VDRL test. Syphilis is effectively treated with penicillin. Pregnant women with syphilis who are allergic to penicillin should undergo inpatient desensitization so that treatment with penicillin will be possible.

TOXOPLASMOSIS

Toxoplasmosis is an infection caused by the protozoan *Toxoplasma gondii*. It is widely distributed in nature, and the domestic cat is a very common host. Approximately one-third of the adult women in the United States have *Toxoplasma* antibodies, which indicates prior infection. *Toxoplasma* is acquired by eating undercooked meat of animals containing infective tissue cysts or by inhaling or ingesting the microorganism excreted in the feces of domestic cats. It is also transmitted from mother to fetus. It has been shown that transmission to the fetus occurs virtually only when women acquire the

169

infection during pregnancy. Women infected before becoming pregnant have virtually no risk of transmitting the disease to their offspring. One exception is immunocompromised patients, including mothers infected with HIV.

Acute *Toxoplasma* infection goes undetected in approximately 90% of cases. The signs and symptoms are so minor and unspecific that patients usually don't seek medical attention. When it is symptomatic, acute toxoplasmosis presents with fever, malaise, and adenopathy, mostly in head and neck. Transmission of *Toxoplasma* to the fetus can cause abortion or infected fetuses with congenital toxoplasmosis. Approximately 50% to 60% of fetuses whose mothers acquire the infection during pregnancy are affected. Three-quarters of them are asymptomatic but show sequelae later in life. Congenital toxoplasmosis can cause chorioretinitis, hydrocephalus, and microcephalus. Congenital infection is more common after maternal infection during the third trimester, but the sequelae are less severe. Serology (presence of antibodies against *Toxoplasma* in the serum) is the best method for diagnosis of maternal toxoplasmosis. Unfortunately, the inaccuracy of available tests and the low prevalence of acute toxoplasmosis in pregnancy make routine screening not recommended in the United States. In countries where maternal toxoplasmosis is more common, routine screening during prenatal visits is mandatory. The American College of Obstetrics and Gynecology recommends that if serologic screening is considered in women of reproductive age, the best time to perform it is prior to pregnancy. If specific antibodies are present, that will indicate prior infection and maternal immunity that will avoid congenital disease. However, this approach is not helpful in cases of absence of antibodies prior to conception. Some in the United States have advocated routine serological screening, suggesting that congenital infection is much more common and is going underdetected because of the lack of routine prenatal testing.

In cases where the diagnosis of acute *Toxoplasma* infection is made early in pregnancy, therapeutic abortion has been recommended. An alternative is treatment with antibiotics. Spiramycin has been widely used in Europe for this purpose. It reduces the frequency of maternal transmission in about 60% of cases. This antibiotic is not currently approved by the Food and Drug Administration (FDA) for this use in the United States. However, it is available to physicians through the FDA on a case-by-case basis. Combinations of other drugs might be more effective, but also more teratogenic in the first trimester.

RUBELLA

Also known as German measles, rubella is caused by a virus. In nonpregnant women and the general population, it is a disease of little consequence.

It is contagious and may present with fever, rash, and neck adenopathy, especially postauricular lymph node enlargement. A large number of cases present without symptoms. Epidemics of rubella have virtually disappeared in developed countries because of routine vaccination during childhood.

In the United States, however, it is estimated that 6% to 25% of women are still susceptible. It has been well documented that rubella acquired during pregnancy has devastating effects on the fetus. One published series of mothers who acquired rubella during pregnancy showed that 4% had spontaneous abortions and another 2% had stillbirths. Of the fetuses that survived, all of them whose mothers were infected before the 11th week had congenital defects; only 36% had such defects when the infection occurred after the 13th week. The clinical manifestation of congenital rubella varies, depending on the timing of maternal infection and the stage of fetal development. It can include eye lesions resulting in blindness, heart disease, deafness, lung abnormalities, and chromosomal abnormalities.

The main preventive measure is vaccination. However, it is not currently recommended shortly before or during pregnancy because the vaccine is made of live virus. Therefore it is very important to establish presence of antibodies (which indicates prior infection) in all women of reproductive age before pregnancy. In cases where antibodies are present, it will be extremely rare for the mother to infect a fetus if reexposed. If antibodies cannot be demonstrated, vaccination is mandatory. The woman should not get pregnant for the next three months.

MEASLES

Measles is a very contagious viral disease that is common during childhood. It has become rare in developed countries because of routine vaccination during childhood. It usually manifests as fever, malaise, rash, pharyngitis, and conjunctivitis. It can be more complicated in adults, and about 3% will develop pneumonia. Pregnant women do not appear to have a more complicated course. There are no conclusive studies about the effects of the virus on the fetus, probably because of the rarity of the disease during pregnancy. There is consensus, however, that measles can cause an increased rate of abortion and premature labor. In a report of fifty-eight pregnancies complicated by measles, 50% of them ended within fourteen days of the onset of measles rash. That included five spontaneous abortions and eleven preterm deliveries. The virus does not appear to be teratogenic, meaning that surviving fetuses will not have an increased risk of malformations.

Measles that is apparent in the first ten days of life is considered congenital. The mortality rate in those cases is around 30%. The mortality rate in premature infants with congenital measles is approximately 50%.

PARVOVIRUS

Human parvoviruses are a group of viruses of which the most common is B19. It causes a disease known as fifth disease, erythema infectiosum, or roseola infantum. It is more common in children, very contagious, and generally mild. It may be asymptomatic or present with facial rash (slapped cheek appearance), fever, and malaise. In adults rash is usually not present, and they more commonly present with fever, arthralgia, and adenopathy. In the United States, 50% to 75% of women of reproductive age are immune, with antibodies in serum.

In cases of primary infection during pregnancy, parvovirus B19 can be transmitted to the fetus through the placenta. Fetal infection can cause spontaneous abortion, intrauterine fetal death, fetal anemia, and gross anemia. It is not clear, however, how frequent these complications are. There are series in the literature showing cases of fetal loss associated with B19 infection, but in most of them the rate of pregnancy loss among women infected during pregnancy was not significantly higher than in the normal population.

The current recommendation is that women exposed to parvovirus during pregnancy should be screened for presence of antibodies. If IgG is present, meaning prior infection, they can be reassured. If IgG is absent and IgM (reflects acute infection) is also absent, they are susceptible and therefore should reduce the risks of exposure. This is especially important for day care workers and schoolteachers. If IgG is absent and IgM is present, the mother should be followed closely with serial ultrasounds to detect any fetal abnormality, including edema.

VARICELLA

The *Varicella zoster* virus causes chickenpox. The disease is common in childhood, and most adult women are immune because of previous infection. There are reports which suggest that chickenpox can be especially severe in pregnancy. Pneumonitis, a serious complication, can present more frequently in pregnant women with chickenpox than in nonpregnant affected adults, thus increasing the chances of fetal complications.

It is well documented that maternal chickenpox during the first 20 weeks of pregnancy will cause congenital varicella syndrome in about 2% of the cases. This syndrome is characterized by fetal malformations, typically bony defects and scarring in limbs, chorioretinitis, or hydronephrosis. There have been cases of spontaneous abortion and fetal death after 20 weeks secondary to in utero *Varicella* infection, but they are rare. In a series of 1,373 pregnant women with chickenpox, only one case of spontaneous abortion at 16 weeks and one case of fetal death at 23 weeks could be proved to be related to in utero *Varicella* infection.

CYTOMEGALOVIRUS

Cytomegalovirus (CMV) is a virus that infects about 80% of the population. After the primary infection the virus becomes latent and periodically is reactivated, meaning that there is not effective lifetime immunity after the first infection. CMV infection is a serious health problem only in immunosupressed people and in fetuses and newborns. Most infections are asymptomatic; in about 15% of the cases the person will present mononucleosis-type symptoms.

CMV can be transmitted to the fetus via the placenta and also through the birth canal, since CMV can infect the uterine cervix. There are no reports that suggest CMV infection in utero can cause spontaneous abortion or fetal death. CMV, however, can cause a congenital infection that has devastating effects on newborns and their families. The syndrome includes intracranial calcifications, chorioretinitis, low birth weight, blindness, deafness, and mental retardation. It can also cause neonatal death.

It is estimated that 0.5% to 2% of all neonates are infected. Of those, 5% to 10% can have neurologic sequelae. Severe disease thus occurs in 1 in every 10,000 to 20,000 newborns. It has been shown that only fetuses from mothers with primary infection are at risk for severe sequelae (in approximately 25% of those cases). Severe sequelae also are more common if the infection occurs during the first trimester. Newborns exposed in utero to recurrent infection have a minor risk of sequelae and probably have no risk of developing mental retardation.

Unfortunately, there is no treatment for maternal infection, nor is there a way to prevent fetuses from becoming infected once the mother acquires the infection. While there is an ongoing investigation to develop an effective vaccine, the only effective way to reduce this public health problem is by prevention. Most experts recommend that women of reproductive age should have their CMV antibody status determined. This will show if a person has been infected, in which case the risk of having a baby with significant sequelae will be very low in the event of a new infection during pregnancy. Women who are CMV-seronegative, and therefore susceptible to primary infection, should be counseled. Once they become pregnant, they should avoid contact with urine and saliva from infants and practice careful hygiene. They should minimize sharing of glasses and other utensils and avoid sexual contact with a partner having evident mononucleosis-like infection, since CMV can be transmitted sexually. If a primary infection is documented during pregnancy and/or if fetal abnormalities consistent with

CMV congenital infection are found, therapeutic termination of the pregnancy should be considered.

LISTERIOSIS

Listeriosis is caused by the bacterium *Listeria monocytogenes*. *Listeria* is usually a food-borne pathogen, often found in contaminated or nonpasteurized dairy products. It can also be isolated from soil, water, sewage, and human feces.

Listeriosis is a rare but catastrophic complication of pregnancy. The infection presents without symptoms or as a febrile illness that can be confused with influenza or other infectious diseases. *Listeria* infection in the mother is spread through the blood to the uterine cavity and the fetus. Although there are no data showing the percentage of fetuses affected, not all fetuses are infected during maternal listeriosis.

The diagnosis is made by isolation of the bacteria in maternal blood, amniotic fluid, or the placenta, or from the fetus in case of fetal infection. Maternal listeriosis causes a high incidence of second and third trimester pregnancy losses. The mortality of neonates born with congenital listeriosis is around 50%. There is now evidence that treating the mother with antibiotic combinations intravenously may prevent perinatal mortality.

SALMONELLOSIS

Salmonella is a bacterium that commonly contaminates poultry and egg products. A major cause of food poisoning, it is characterized by diarrhea, abdominal pain, cramping, and fever. Usually it is a self-limited infection requiring no antibiotic treatment. There are two major groups of *Salmonella* species: *typhy* and nontyphoid. *Salmonella typhy* spreads through the blood and causes a more serious disease, typhoid. In pregnant women typhoid causes pregnancy loss in around 80% of the cases if not treated with appropriate antibiotics. The diagnosis is made by isolation of the bacteria in blood or stools or by serologic testing. The incidence of pregnancy losses caused by nontyphoid *Salmonella* is probably much less. However, there are no data in the literature to fully illustrate the effect of this species on pregnancy.

SHIGELLOSIS

Shigella is another relatively common cause of food poisoning, characterized by bloody stools, abdominal cramping, and general toxicity. Like most cases of salmonellosis, it is a self-limited infection and does not require antimicrobial treatment. The main risk that shigellosis poses to pregnant women is by producing dehydration and electrolyte imbalances secondary to intense secretory diarrhea.

LYME DISEASE

Lyme disease is caused by a spirochete that is transmitted through the bite of ticks. Initially the disease is localized, causing a characteristic skin rash, a influenza-type illness, and lymph node enlargement. If not treated, the infection may affect the heart, joints, and central nervous system. The diagnosis is usually made on clinical findings. Serologic testing (presence of specific antibodies in serum) is also useful. Lyme disease is usually treated with antibiotics, with better results if treated earlier. The consequences of Lyme disease in pregnancy are not totally known. There are a few reports of pregnant women contracting Lyme disease and delivering dead fetuses. In these cases the spirochetes were isolated from different fetal organs, suggesting that Lyme disease may have had a role in those pregnancy losses. More recently, however, a larger series of pregnant women in an area endemic for Lyme disease showed that maternal infection was not associated with fetal death, preterm delivery, or malformation. Until more conclusive data are available, preventive intervention, specifically against tick bites, is the best way to avoid Lyme disease.

HEPATITIS

Hepatitis, inflammation of the liver, can occur as a result of many different insults to the liver. Here we will focus on hepatitis caused by viral infection, which in general is the most common form. Viral hepatitis is the most common liver disease in pregnant women. Currently there are five different viruses that can cause hepatitis: A, B, C, D and E. This discussion will cover the most common ones, hepatitis A and B.

Hepatitis A is usually benign in well nourished people. The main concerns during the disease are to rest and to maintain good nutrition. There are no data suggesting that hepatitis A increases the risk of spontaneous abortion more than any other febrile disease. Nor does it increase the risks of fetal malformation. There may be a slightly higher risk of preterm labor during an acute maternal infection. The major impact on the mother and fetus could be caused by hepatitis B. There is no clear evidence that the hepatitis B virus is transmitted through the placenta to the fetus. The major mechanism of fetal infection appears to be ingestion by the newborn of infected maternal blood and fluids during delivery. Approximately 80% to 90% of newborns of mothers who develop acute hepatitis B in the third trimester acquire the virus. A small percentage of these develop fulminant hepatitis and die during the first few months. Another small group may not get infected. The rest, about 80%, will become chronic carriers and will be at a higher risk of developing cirrhosis and liver cancer. The incidence of spontaneous abortion in first trimester patients with acute hepatitis B is increased.

When it is contracted during the third trimester, there is an increased incidence of preterm labor. Teratogenic effect has never been demonstrated.

GONORRHEA

Gonorrhea, a disease caused by the bacterium *Neisseria gonnorhoeae*, is a relatively common sexually transmitted disease. Most of the time the infection is limited to the genitals, especially the cervix. In women gonorrhea can be asymptomatic, hence the importance of routine screening especially in pregnant women. If the infection is not diagnosed and treated, it increases the risk of spontaneous abortion, most likely secondary to cervical inflammation during the first trimester. It also increases the risk of preterm labor and infections of the uterine cavity.

HUMAN IMMUNODEFICIENCY VIRUS (HIV)

Transmission of human immunodeficiency virus (HIV) from mother to infant is well established. Possible routes of transmission include the placenta, contact with contaminated fluid and blood during the delivery, and postnatally in association with breast-feeding. The frequency of each mechanism is not clear, however. Approximately 10% to 40% of infants born to seropositive women become infected. The average in most series is about 30%. The majority of infants with congenitally acquired HIV die within the first two years of life.

Initially it was thought that HIV infection did not interfere with the pregnancy outcome. Recently, however, a report of a series of HIV-infected mothers showed an increased rate of spontaneous abortion. The rate was higher in mothers who had developed the acquired immunodeficiency syndrome (AIDS) than in asymptomatic mothers.

The rate of HIV transmission during pregnancy can be successfully diminished with antiretroviral therapy. Treatment with zidovudine starting between 18 and 34 weeks and continued until delivery can decrease the percentage of infected newborns to below 10%. Some authors recommend delivery by cesarean section to avoid contact of the fetus with contaminated blood and fluid during passage through the birth canal. Breast-feeding should also be avoided because of virus transmission through breast milk.

HERPES

Herpes simplex virus (HSV) causes what has become one of the most common sexually transmitted diseases. The first episode, known as the primary infection, is usually more severe. It is characterized by multiple fluid-filled lesions in the genitalia associated with extreme pain and discomfort. It is also commonly associated with flulike symptoms. After the first episode, the virus stays latent and the person remains without symptoms. The recurrences are typically milder and shorter.

Unfortunately, the benefit of currently known antiviral medications is to shorten the active episode; the virus cannot be totally eliminated. Transmission of HSV from mother to fetus can have catastrophic consequences. The virus is rarely transmitted through the placenta. The fetus almost always acquires it by passage through the birth canal, or the virus my ascend through ruptured membranes and contaminate the fetus. If the herpetic neonatal infection is localized, the outcome is generally good. However, in disseminated neonatal infection the mortality is 50% to 60%. Interestingly, the risks of neonatal infection are approximately 50% in cases in which the mother has a primary infection, versus approximately 5% during recurrent infections.

The evidence of the effect of herpes infection on the pregnancy outcome is controversial. A number of reports have suggested that first-episode infection is associated with some increased risk of spontaneous abortion. However, these results were not reproduced in several other investigations. There is more agreement that it increases the risk of premature delivery by 30% to 50%. There are no data to suggest bad pregnancy outcome as a result of recurrent infection. If herpes infection is diagnosed during labor, the current recommendation is to deliver by cesarean section. This is to avoid further contact of the newborn with contaminated maternal tissue. It has been shown that treating mothers known to have had herpes in the past with acyclovir (an antiviral) from the 36th week until delivery will effectively reduce the recurrences and neonatal infections, and avoid cesarean sections.

CHLAMYDIA

Lower genital tract infection with *Chlamydia trachomatis* is currently the most commonly diagnosed sexually transmitted disease. It has been estimated that 20% to 40% of sexually active women in the United States have been infected with chlamydia. The infection can be asymptomatic, or it can cause mucopurulent vaginal discharge and pain. When untreated, it can ascend to upper genital organs and cause pelvic inflammatory disease (PID). PID is rare in pregnancy, but when it occurs, it can cause pregnancy loss in approximately 50% of the cases. Chlamydia and gonorrhea are the two most common causes of PID.

The effects of chlamydia infection on the newborn are well characterized. Usually, if the mother's genital tract is colonized, the newborn will acquire the infection during delivery. Conjunctivitis develops in up to 50% of infected newborns. This complication can lead to blindness if not treated. Between 10% and 20% develop pneumonia. What is more debatable is the role of maternal chlamydial infection in the pregnancy outcome. Some reports suggest that chlamydial infection is strongly associated with spontaneous abortion, preterm labor, and uterine infection. However, other investigations were unable to prove any relationship. More recently, it has been shown that only women with evidence of recent infection are at a higher risk of premature rupture of membranes and preterm labor.

Under current obstetrical practice, all pregnant women are routinely checked for chlamydia infection early in the pregnancy. If the culture results are positive, treatment with antibiotics is prescribed.

MYCOPLASMA

Mycoplasma species that colonize the female genital tract include *M. hominis* and *Ureaplasma urealyticum*. These microorganism probably are sexually transmitted. They have been cultured from the genital tract in 15% to 75% of sexually active women, being more prevalent in women with more sexual partners.

Mycoplasma colonization has been suggested, not without controversy, as a cause of recurrent spontaneous abortion, stillbirth, and preterm delivery. Several studies have found *Mycoplasma* in fetal material in significantly larger numbers of spontaneous abortions compared to induced abortions. Similarly, several investigators have reported a higher incidence of genital colonization with *Mycoplasma* in women experiencing repeated spontaneous abortions compared to normal women. These results may suggest an association between *Mycoplasma* genital colonization and spontaneous pregnancy loss. These studies, however, are not conclusive enough to establish that *Mycoplasma* indeed infected the fetus, causing its death; it is also possible that the fetus died from other causes and then became more susceptible to infection by ascending microorganisms. *Mycoplasma* has also been implicated as a cause of preterm birth. However a recent multicenter report showed that *Mycoplasma* colonization was not correlated with preterm labor, preterm delivery, or low birth weight. Similarly, studies investigating the role of routine *Mycoplasma* cultures and even treatment with antibiotics before pregnancy in women with recurrent pregnancy loss have not consistently found that treatment to be beneficial. The presence of genital *Mycoplasma* does not appear to cause serious newborn illnesses, even after contact during the birth process.

In summary, current scientific data do not support the hypothesis that *Mycoplasma* colonization of the genital tract increases risk of pregnancy loss, nor do they recommend routine cultures for *Mycoplasma* or treatment with antibiotics.

GROUP B STREPTOCOCCAL INFECTION

Group B *Streptococcus* (GBS) is a bacterium that commonly colonizes the female genital tract. Between 10% and 30% of pregnant women are colonized with GBS in the vaginal or rectal area. This organism has been recognized as a cause of illnesses and death in newborn infants and in parturient women.

In pregnant women GBS can cause urinary tract infection, infection of the uterine cavity (especially after a cesarean section), and infection of the surgical wound. In newborns GBS is responsible for infection of various organs (meningitis, pneumonia, cellulitis, etc.) that can spread, causing sepsis and death. The risk of sepsis in the United States is about 1.8 per 1,000 live births. The mortality rate is between 5% and 20%.

Early reports suggested that GBS genital colonization was associated with an increased risk of stillbirth, preterm rupture of membranes, and premature deliveries. However, data to support this association have been inconsistent. What is more accepted is the association between presence of GBS bacteriuria (presence of bacteria in urine) and preterm delivery. Bacteriuria is an indicator of heavy genital colonization. In other words, women who are heavily colonized with GBS are at a higher risk of preterm delivery. Women lightly colonized are probably at the same risk as women not colonized. The main route of neonatal contamination thus is passage through the birth canal. Another important route is through ruptured membranes that allow the bacteria to ascend to the uterine cavity.

Besides heavy colonization, there are other risk factors that influence the rate of newborn GBS infection. These include rupture of membranes for more than eighteen hours before delivery, preterm birth, and maternal chorioamnionitis (infection of the uterus and pregnancy-related tissues). Fortunately, GBS is very susceptible to antibiotic therapy. The main issue is who receives it and when to give it in order to prevent neonatal infection.

Several national agencies have developed guidelines for administering antibiotics to pregnant women close to or in labor. These are basically based on the presence of risk factors. It is well established that timely administration of antibiotics to colonized women will effectively prevent both neonatal complications and postpartum infections.

Renal Agenesis and Hypoplastic Lung Syndrome

Ande L. Karimu, MD, PhD

Renal agenesis and hypoplastic lung syndrome are congenital malformations of neonates involving the kidneys and the lungs, respectively (i.e., the newborns are born with these disorders). There are both inherited and environmental factors in the causation of the malformations. Often both conditions coexist as part of multiple congenital malformations.

RENAL AGENESIS

Renal agenesis is the complete absence of the kidney(s). The kidneys are the organs that filter waste products from the blood, eliminating them as urine.

Under normal circumstances there are two kidneys in the human. Absence of the kidney can be unilateral or bilateral. If it is unilateral, only one kidney is absent; if it is bilateral, both kidneys are absent. Unilateral absence of a kidney is compatible with life, whereas bilateral absence of the kidneys is not.

DEVELOPMENT OF THE KIDNEYS

The kidneys are parts of the urinary system. Other members of the system include the ureters, the bladder, and the urethra. The urinary system develops in close association with the genital organs. The kidneys develop in three main stages: the pronephros, the mesonephros, and the metanephros (*nephros* means kidney). The pronephros are nonfunctional and soon degenerate, being replaced by the mesonephros, which function for a short time before they are in turn replaced by the metanephros, the definitive kidneys. The metanephros begin to develop in the fifth week of intrauterine life. Urine formation begins about the end of the first trimester (the 12th week of pregnancy) and continues for the rest of the pregnancy. The urine produced by the fetus is secreted into the amniotic cavity and forms part of the amniotic fluid. In the fetus, the placenta is the main organ of excretion, so the kidneys don't need to be functional as excretory organs during intrauterine life. However, they must be ready to assume their excretory functions at birth.

Earlier in pregnancy the kidneys are located in the pelvis, but by the ninth week of pregnancy the kidneys have attained their final position in the abdomen. For this reason, it is often observed that the kidneys have various sources of blood supply during development that gradually degenerate as the kidneys ascend to the abdominal cavity. Not surprisingly, the adult kidneys sometimes have an aberrant blood supply due to their migratory development.

Complete absence of the kidneys (bilateral renal agenesis) results when both metanephric buds fail to develop, while unilateral renal agenesis results from one-sided metanephric bud absence.

CLINICAL FEATURES

During prenatal life, renal agenesis can be diagnosed with ultrasound examination that reveals oligohydramnios (reduced amniotic fluid volume) and absence of the kidney(s). In most U.S. centers, targeted ultrasound for detailed anatomical survey of the fetus is carried out around the 18th–20th week of gestation. At this time, based on the reduced fluid volume, clinical suspicion is high; detailed anatomical survey will reveal the absence of the kidney(s). However, ultrasound examination may not always reveal the absence of kidneys due to oligohydramnios. Moreover, adrenal tissues may be confused with renal tissue. In this situation, serial evaluation over four to six hours to confirm absence of urine production, as demonstrated by failure to visualize the fetal bladder, may be very useful in establishing the diagnosis with certainty.

Absence of one kidney is compatible with life; the other kidney enlarges to compensate for the absent one. For this reason, as adults we can donate one kidney and still carry on effectively with the remaining kidney. In the unlikely event that an absent kidney is not diagnosed before birth, it may be diagnosed in adulthood as an incidental finding during imaging studies of the abdomen for some other reason.

With regard to bilateral renal agenesis, the fetus is stillborn in more than 40% of cases, and the majority of infants born alive usually die within four hours. The characteristic features of these infants, called Potter's facies, include redundant and dehydrated skin, wide-set eyes, a prominent fold arising at the inner canthus of each eye, parrot beak nose, receding chin, large, low-set ears with deficient auricular cartilage, absent urine output, and nonpalpable kidneys. Death shortly after birth is attributed to either pulmonary hypoplasia or renal failure. Other congenital anomalies associated with bilateral renal agenesis include absence of the urinary bladder, bilateral pulmonary hypoplasia, genital organ abnormalities (e.g., absence of the vas deferens and the seminal vesicles in males and the uterus and upper vagina in females), anal atresia, absence of the rectum and the sigmoid colon, esophageal and duodenal atresia, single umbilical artery, and major abnormalities of the lower limbs.

MANAGEMENT OF RENAL AGENESIS

The best management approach is taking preventive measures, as much as possible, to prevent congenital malformations from occurring. For instance, a pregnant woman with uncontrolled diabetes mellitus is prone to having a baby with congenital malformations including renal agenesis. Adequate control of diabetes in pregnancy will reduce the likelihood of this malformation.

HYPOPLASTIC LUNG SYNDROME

This is underdevelopment of the lungs. It commonly results from abnormal development of the diaphragm, a muscular structure that separates the thoracic (chest) cavity from the abdominal cavity. It also may occur as one of multiple congenital anomalies affecting a fetus that include renal agenesis, urinary tract outflow obstruction, extra-amniotic fetal development, and thoracic dystrophies. Other associations include intrauterine central nervous system damage sufficient to decrease fetal breathing movement, trisomy 21, erythroblastosis fetalis (fetal isoimmunization), and certain drugs (e.g., ACE inhibitors). Abnormal development of the diaphragm is the more common cause, and this is amenable to surgical correction soon after birth. I will therefore describe development of the diaphragm in more detail and how its malformation may result in hypoplastic lung syndrome.

DEVELOPMENT OF THE DIAPHRAGM

The diaphragm develops from four structures: the septum transversum, pleuroperitoneal membranes, dorsal mesentery of the esophagus, and the body wall. The septum transversum is the part of the embryonic mesoderm that separates the pericardial cavity from the gut. It forms the definitive central tendon of the diaphragm. The central tendon is a trifoliate aponeurotic structure that fuses with the pericardium of the heart. The pleuroperitoneal membranes separate the pleural and the peritoneal cavities. The pleural cavity contains the lungs and the peritoneal cavity contains the abdominal organs. By the sixth week of intrauterine life, the pleuroperitoneal membranes usually fuse with the dorsal mesentery of the esophagus and the septum transversum, thus effectively separating the pleural and the peritoneal cavities (i.e., the chest and the abdomen). In fetal life, the pleuroperitoneal membranes represent a large portion of the diaphragm, but are a small part of the definitive diaphragm. The dorsal mesentery of the esophagus is a double layer of peritoneum that forms the median portion of the diaphragm. Two slips of muscles, the right and left crura, arise from the lumbar vertebrae and grow into the dorsal mesentery around the 9th to 12th week of intrauterine life.

The body wall is the most peripheral part of the diaphragm. The developing fetal lungs and pleural cavity usually invade the body wall. At this time the body wall divides into two layers, with the inner layer forming the definitive peripheral rim of the diaphragm. During development of the diaphragm, the septum transversum, the first indication of the developing diaphragm, lies in the cervical (neck) region, opposite the third to the fifth cervical somites. During the 5th week of development, the muscle cells from these somites migrate into the developing diaphragm, taking their nerves (phrenic nerves) with them from the cervical region. As the diaphragm migrates to its final location in the thorax, the phrenic nerve accompanies it, thus traversing almost 30 centimeters.

Congenital Diaphragmatic Hernia

This is a relatively common congenital malformation of the diaphragm occurring in 1 of 2,000 newborns. It results from a defect in the posterolateral region of the diaphragm. Congenital posterolateral defect of the diaphragm is due to nonfusion of the pleuroperitoneal membranes with the septum transversum and the dorsal mesentery of the esophagus. It is usually unilateral, occurring commonly on the left side. The reason for the left-sided preponderance is due to the early closure of the right pleuroperitoneal membrane secondary to the presence of the bulky embryonic liver on the right side. Normally, the pleuroperitoneal membranes fuse with the other diaphragmatic components by the 7th week of intrauterine life. If a pleuroperitoneal membrane is unfused by the time the intestine returns from the umbilical cord to the abdomen, around the 10th week of intrauterine life, the intestine usually passes into the thorax. The spleen and stomach may also herniate into the thorax. At birth, the thoracic intestines usually dilate with swallowed air, compromising the functions of the heart and lungs. The mediastinum and its contents, including the heart, are usually displaced to the right and the lungs are hypoplastic (underdeveloped). Normally during pregnancy the lungs are filled with fluids that help to maintain their volume. However, because of compression from intra-abdominal organs, the lungs are not able to accumulate enough fluid to maintain the requisite volume; hence their underdevelopment.

Diagnosis of Diaphragmatic Hernia

At birth the newborn will demonstrate evidence of respiratory distress syndrome with dyspnea, tachypnea, cyanosis, tachycardia, and so on. The lungs may be dull to percussion due to nonexpansion after birth, and air entry to the lungs will be remarkably reduced on auscultation. Imaging studies of the chest and abdomen will reveal the presence of abdominal organs in the thoracic cavity.

Clinical Management

The immediate goals are to return the abdominal organs to their definitive positions in the abdomen and to close the diaphragmatic defects. Once the hernia is reduced, the affected lungs usually expand with aeration and ultimately achieve their normal size.

CONCLUSION

The etiology of congenital anomalies is usually multifactorial; both genetic and environmental factors play a role. Some of the causative factors are amenable to control by preventive measures. Some examples are the recommended intake of folic acid in pregnancy to reduce the likelihood of malformations of the brain and tight glucose control to ameliorate possible renal malformation. Others include avoidance of medications such as ACE inhibitors during pregnancy and avoidance of over-the-counter medications of unproven safety. Until we can determine with certainty the etiology of congenital anomalies, the best that can be done is mainly preventive. In any case, prevention is better than cure, and certainly cheaper.

Postterm Pregnancy

Rotimi Odutayo, MD, MRCOG, and Kunle Odunsi, MD, PhD, MRCOG

In 1902 Ballantyne[47] made the first reference to postterm pregnancy in modern obstetrics. In 1954 Clifford[48] more succinctly described a syndrome found in infants born after the expected date of delivery that in many respects resembled intrauterine growth retardation; there was often thick meconium staining of the amniotic fluid and signs of fetal distress during labor in these postmature infants. Hasseljo[49] and Lanman[50] also showed that there was an increased risk of intrapartum death associated with prolonged pregnancy, and a study from Scandinavia confirmed that prolonged pregnancy was associated with an increased risk of perinatal death.[51] An observational study from Dublin examined the risks of postmaturity in 6,301 pregnancies delivered at 42 weeks.[52] In the postmature pregnancies, intrapartum stillbirth was four times, and neonatal death three times, more common than in women delivered at term, and early neonatal seizures were ten times more common. Crowley[53] compared the outcomes of labor in 247 women delivered after 42 weeks with 247 matched controls delivered between 37 and 42 weeks: meconium-stained amniotic fluid occurred twice as often in the postmature women and the need for fetal blood sampling was four times as common.

Prolonged pregnancy has gained prominence in the last decade as a probable high-risk condition after widespread use of antenatal testing. This notoriety has developed more as a consequence of the inability to find the appropriate sensitive antenatal test than of the acceptance of its truly life-threatening condition for some fetuses. This point is clearly observed when one reviews publications stating that perinatal mortality is the same in prolonged and in term gestations.[54]

EPIDEMIOLOGY

The World Health Organization (WHO)[55] and International Federation of Gynecology and Obstetrics (FIGO)[56] have defined prolonged pregnancy as 42 completed weeks or more (lasting more than two weeks beyond the confirmed expected date of delivery). "Postterm pregnancy," "prolonged pregnancy," "postdate pregnancy," and "after-term pregnancy" are used synonymously. They are therefore used interchangeably in this review.

The accurate determination of the expected day of confinement is a key issue in the antenatal and neonatal periods for both clinical obstetrics and research. It has profound personal, social, and medical implications for the expectant mother. There are problems in estimating the incidence of prolonged pregnancy, not just because of differing definitions but also because of incomplete recording of pregnancies, differences between hospital and population surveys, differing policies for induction of labor, and varying proportions of women with uncertain dates.[57] Between 4% and 14% (average 10%) of women are prepared to reach 42 weeks' gestation, and 2% to 7% (average 4%) to reach 43 weeks' gestation, depending on the population studied.[58] There have been suggestions that the duration of normal pregnancy may be related to maternal characters, such as height,[59] parity,[60] and race.[61] In studies where conception has been estimated from basal body temperature charts,[62] and ultrasound measurements,[63] it has been shown that the error in menstrual dating is heavily skewed to the right (i.e., there is a tendency to overestimate gestation).

In spite of all this evidence, the last menstrual period (LMP) continues to be the basis for estimating the duration of pregnancy. Often this is unknown, in which case gestational age may be estimated by ultrasonographic measurements of fetal parameters such as the crown–rump length[64] until about 12 weeks, and the biparietal diameter (BPD)[65] from about 14 to 22 weeks' gestation. There is no uniform dating policy when both a valid LMP and ultrasonographic dates are available. In practice, many obstetrics and ultrasound departments follow a seven-, ten-, or fourteen-day rule[66] whereby preference is given to menstrual dates if they are within seven, ten, or fourteen days, respectively, from the ultrasonographic estimate. However, the random error in dating by ultrasound measurement of the BPD in the second trimester has been estimated at 3.2 days[67] and, unlike menstrual dates, this error is normally distributed.[68] It is now clear that even if menstrual dates are considered certain, there is no advantage in taking them into consideration for calculating the expected date of delivery if a dating ultrasonography result is available. Dating by ultrasonographic biometry in the first half of pregnancy results in a more accurate prediction of the delivery date than using menstrual date alone or in combination with ultrasonography.[69]

DIAGNOSIS

It is obvious from the available literature that the correct diagnosis of postdate pregnancy is very difficult. The WHO definition[70] of term pregnancy as 259 to 294 days from LMP was based on statistical data derived from menstrual dates. It has been shown that even if the LMP is recalled with accuracy, it will not be a reliable indicator of the actual date of conception. This is because the onset of ovulation within the menstrual cycle is erratic and may vary from one cycle to the next.[71] Dating policies have important clinical implications.

Because of unreliability of the menstrual dating[72] and the fact that most obstetric units induce labor for postmaturity and postterm based on the menstrual history, this method of historical diagnosis will result in a high proportion of women having unnecessary induction of labor for postmaturity. Ultrasonography in the first half of pregnancy will reduce the percentage of pregnancies classified as postterm by WHO definition (42 weeks) from 11.5 to 3.5 (i.e., by 70%).

Mothers, midwives, and physicians are often uncertain as to which date should be used, and this may lead to considerable parental confusion. A uniform dating policy would reduce much of the uncertainty in pregnancy dating.[73] The available evidence strongly supports the view that dating by ultrasonography alone is the most accurate method for predicting EDC. Confinement occurred on the day predicted in 3.6% if EDC was based on the LMP and in 4.3% if it was based on the ultrasound scan. Delivery took place within seven days of the EDC in 49.5% cases when LMP alone was used and in 55.2% if ultrasonography alone was used. If this margin of error was widened to 10 days, the corresponding figures were 64.1% and 70.3%.[74]

FETAL SURVEILLANCE

We now have available many forms of testing to follow the well-being of the postterm fetus while it is still in utero. There is considerable uncertainty, however, as to how well these tests measure fetal compromise and how effective treatment is when these tests are used in management. Whatever form of testing is chosen, it is important to remember that the condition of the fetus can change quickly. Thus, monitoring should be at frequent intervals, and none of the tests are immune from false positives or false negatives.[75] Perinatal mortality rates (excluding lethal congenital anomalies) have been reported to be as low as 1.1–1.2 per 1,000 with close surveillance.[76] Postterm perinatal deaths continue to occur, however, some of them within twenty-four to forty-eight hours of normal fetal assessment. Furthermore, despite current techniques of fetal surveillance, there continue to be reports of higher risks of fetal and neonatal morbidity and operative delivery with postterm, compared to term, pregnancy.[77] The various available tests are described below.

Fetal Movement Counting

Fetal movement counting has been a popular method of fetal surveillance because it allows the mother to participate actively in the evaluation of her baby's health.[78] Although one small controlled trial suggested that this form of monitoring might be effective in decreasing the perinatal mortality rate, a larger trial undertaken in many centers in Europe and the United States showed no beneficial effect.[79] Neither of these trials focused on postterm pregnancy. In the Canadian Multicenter Postterm Pregnancy Trial, women allocated to the expectant group were asked to count daily until they counted six movements, or for two hours (whichever took less time). If after two hours the woman had felt fewer than six movements, she was to contact her obstetrician for further evaluation. Only 2.2% (38/1,707) of women reported decreased fetal movements. The two women in the trial with still-births (excluding lethal anomalies) did not report decreased fetal movement counts.[80]

Amniotic Fluid Volume

The volume of amniotic fluid has been estimated to decrease by 150–170ml per week after 42 weeks of pregnancy.[81] More recent investigations using real-time ultrasound confirm decreasing amniotic fluid as pregnancies continue past 41 weeks.[82] The reason for this decrease is not completely understood, but may be due to decreased fetal urine production.[83] Amniotic fluid volume as assessed by ultrasound has been evaluated in blind and un-blinded studies in postterm pregnancies, and there is now good evidence that postterm pregnancies with no or low volumes of amniotic fluid are at higher risk of adverse perinatal outcome than pregnancies with a normal amount of amniotic fluid.[84] Low volumes of amniotic fluid, assessed by ul-trasound, in postterm pregnancy have been defined as occurring when the largest pocket of amniotic fluid is less than 3cm in depth, when the sum of the depth of the largest pocket of amniotic fluid in each of four quadrants of the uterus is less than 5cm (amniotic fluid index),[85] or when the product of the length x depth of the largest pocket is less than 60cm. This test is currently considered one of the most sensitive for postterm fetal surveillance and has been used as part of expectant management in five of the random-ized controlled trials of induction of labor compared to expectant manage-ment in postterm pregnancy.[86]

Amnioscopy/Amniocentesis for Assessing the Presence of Meconium

It is known that postterm pregnancies are more frequently complicated by meconium staining of the amniotic fluid than are term pregnancies, and that meconium staining of the amniotic fluid is associated with higher risks of adverse perinatal outcome.[87] It is not unreasonable to suggest, therefore, that amnioscopy or amniocentesis might be a good screening test for fetal compromise in postterm pregnancies. In fact, two randomized controlled trials comparing induction of labor with expectant management have used amnioscopy as part of the surveillance for expectant management.[88] One trial that assessed the effectiveness of weekly amniocentesis (and induction of labor if meconium was present) in postterm pregnancies did not find this better than a program of weekly contraction tests.[89]

Contraction Stress Tests

Some authors have reported on the use of contraction stress tests as a method of fetal surveillance in postterm pregnancy. Both nipple stimulation and intravenous oxytocin have been used as mechanisms for inducing contractions. In some populations the test results appear to correlate with outcome, and some obstetricians prefer this test method of fetal surveillance. The disadvantages are that it takes time to administer and, in the case of the oxytocin challenge test, requires an intravenous infusion.

Nonstress Test

The nonstress test has been a popular method of fetal surveillance for postterm pregnancies.[90] Abnormal test results (nonreactivity and decelerations) have been associated with higher risks of adverse perinatal outcome.[91] Although the test is easy to administer and was used in seven of eleven randomized controlled trials of induction of labor in postterm pregnancy, there is evidence to suggest that it is not an effective method of fetal surveillance. The overview of randomized trials of nonstress testing in the Oxford Database of Perinatal Trials indicates that this testing may result in a higher, rather than a lower, risk of perinatal death because of false reassurance.[92]

Biophysical Profile

The biophysical profile is one of the most popular methods of fetal surveillance for postterm pregnancies. The profile is performed using real-time ultrasound and consists of four distinct measures—fetal breathing, fetal movement, fetal tone, and amniotic fluid volume—with or without the nonstress test. Many who use this as the primary method of fetal surveillance in postterm pregnancy consider the amniotic fluid volume to be the most important measure of the biophysical profile for assessing fetal well-being and, if this one aspect is abnormal, consideration should be given to expediting delivery.

Doppler Ultrasound

Doppler ultrasound of the fetal vessels is the most recent addition to the armamentarium of fetal surveillance for postterm pregnancy. Some studies suggest that it may help to identify pregnancies at higher risk of adverse outcome,[93] whereas others have not found this form of testing to be particularly helpful.[94]

Hormonal Tests

Hormonal tests, such as those for serum or urinary estriols or serum human placental lactogen, have been used to monitor postterm pregnancies. These methods of surveillance are no longer very popular, perhaps more because of their cost and the time required to obtain a result, than because of false diagnoses.

MANAGEMENT

The management of postterm pregnancy that is otherwise uncomplicated is controversial. Central to this controversy is whether the fetus is at increasing risk of deterioration as the pregnancy advances. One management option available for consideration is "active management," when pregnancy is terminated by induction of labor after 41 weeks of gestation. Cervical ripening agents such as prostaglandins[95] are used to prepare the cervix and, if necessary, oxytocin and amniotomy are also used. The other popular option is "expectant management," in which the pregnancy is allowed to progress to 42 weeks and beyond. Labor is induced only if the cervix is well effaced or dilated, or both, or if fetal compromise occurs. The fetal condition is evaluated by various techniques.

Postterm pregnancy has historically been considered a risk factor for adverse perinatal outcome. Before the introduction of fetal surveillance techniques, prolonged pregnancy was associated with a twofold to tenfold increase in the incidence of fetal distress in labor.[96] Induction of labor emerged as a means of reducing perinatal risks in the prolonged pregnancy.

The development and application of modern techniques of fetal assessment have been associated with a reduction in perinatal risk in prolonged pregnancies. In thirteen studies between 1978 and 1987 in which antenatal fetal surveillance was used for follow-up of postterm pregnancies, the risk of perinatal mortality was similar to that of pregnancies delivered at term.[97] Such reports demonstrated that expectant management of postterm pregnancy was an acceptable alternative to induction of labor. However, several studies have suggested that in spite of modern monitoring techniques, the postterm fetus remains at risk for certain perinatal morbidity, such as meconium aspiration, fetal distress in labor, and large body size with its attendant complications.[98] These findings have rekindled the controversy surrounding the optimal management of prolonged pregnancy. In response, prospective randomized trials using contemporary management schemes have compared induction and expectant management in prolonged pregnancy.[99] These trials have yielded conflicting results that have been attributed to differences in patient selection (ripe vs. unripe cervix at entry), methods of labor induction (PGE2 [Prostaglandin E2] with or without oxytocin, amniotomy or stripping of the membranes) and to techniques of antenatal fetal surveillance.

Doubts have been expressed about the value of induction of labor in prolonged pregnancy, mainly that it may result in more operative intervention without necessarily preventing fetal hypoxia and perinatal death from asphyxia. Furthermore, there is a perception among obstetricians that women do not want induction of labor, which may stem from the outcry in the lay press in the 1970s against induction. Thus, in many maternity units induction rates have been falling. This controversy has been partly resolved by the results of sixteen randomized trials, a meta-analysis of which provides clear answers to many of the questions concerning induction of labor.

In conclusion, the available data suggest that induction of labor should be recommended to women with certain dates at 41-plus weeks' gestation, for it will reduce the likelihood of perinatal mortality and of cesarean section for fetal distress.

SHOULD INDUCTION OF LABOR BE ROUTINE? IS IT COST-EFFECTIVE?

From the foregoing, the following conclusions can be deduced. First, contrary to what many obstetricians believe, induction of labor for prolonged pregnancy does not increase the likelihood of cesarean section; rather, it decreases it. Second, the risk of fetal distress from uteroplacental insufficiency due to prolonged pregnancy can be reduced by induction of labor, even to the point of preventing perinatal death from asphyxia. The available evidence suggests that although cesarean sections may be few with induction of labor at 40 weeks, this is offset by an increase in instrumental vaginal delivery. There is little justification for a policy of routine induction of labor at such a relatively early gestation even though perinatal mortality is lowest at 40 weeks' gestation.

Should one recommend induction of labor at 41-plus weeks' gestation to all women with certain dates? Despite the evidence from eleven randomized trials, some obstetricians may not be convinced. The perinatal mortality with induction of labor at 41-plus weeks is 0.3 per 1,000 (1 death in 2,905 cases) and in the control group is 2.5 per 1,000 (7 deaths in 2,822 cases). Thus, in order to prevent one perinatal death, one would have to induce as many as 460 women at 41-plus weeks' gestation. If the reduction in cesarean section rates in a particular maternity unit is 20%, 460 inductions would result in thirteen fewer cesarean sections, hardly a huge saving! Thus a big increase in induction of labor would have to be undertaken in order to secure a comparatively modest gain.

The result of the Canadian Multicenter Postterm Pregnancy Trial and of the meta-analysis, combined with the significant difference in cost between the two strategies (active vs. expectant management) unambiguously supports the induction strategy as a "win-win" alternative in the management of postterm pregnancies. That is, an induction management policy produces better outcome at a lower cost.[100] These findings also support recommendations that induction of labor should be offered to women with pregnancies of 41 or more weeks.[101] More research is needed to determine the most effective methods of induction (e.g., medication, nipple stimulation, stripping or sweeping of the membranes, or mechanical methods).

WOMEN'S VIEWS ABOUT MANAGEMENT OPTIONS

The controversy surrounding the management of prolonged pregnancy has reached a critical point. The available data point to the fact that a huge increase in induction of labor secures only a modest gain. Research on women's views, however, is reassuring. Cardozo[102] asked women, after delivery, to clarify their satisfaction with their treatment allocation into three categories. Dissatisfaction was not associated with treatment allocation, but was strongly associated with operative delivery, regardless of treatment allocation. The study by Roberts et al.[103] showed that the majority of women preferred induction.

REFLECTIONS

One stone casts one shadow
Which cradles the secrets of eternity.
Interred, remains but the bones of your children,
For their flesh and their spirit,
Like the seeds of ancient wildflowers,
Have dissolved into the earth to become one with all humanity.
Nothing will live longer.[1]

We are a society of communicators. Through our speech and literature we portray ourselves, just as paint applied to canvas forms a portrait. We should not underestimate the influence of our words, for they are empowering. In a moment they can help; in less time they can hurt. They can bring peace, and they can create turmoil. A few simple words in an appropriate situation can have inordinate influence. I recently received a note from a father who just had lost his prematurely born daughter to the condition called twin-to-twin transfusion syndrome. One twin died in utero and the remaining twin was born at 25 weeks, gravely ill and on life support systems in the Newborn Intensive Care Unit. After a brave but futile struggle, she, too, died. Her father contacted me from England, asking if I could suggest some words to read at the memorial service for his children. I sent a few lines to these bereaved parents:

Let us not succumb to winter's portent,
the solstice of our darkest hour . . .

In their reply I learned that they will place these words upon the headstone of their twins' grave and will read another poem of mine at their memorial service. Needless to say, I was quite humbled by this use of my

193

poetry. I intend for my words to comfort, and it may take several, if not hundreds, of contacts before they serve such purpose. But when they do, I know that by benefiting just one family, their purpose has been served. I write each poem to reach one family at a time. Since I do not expect a multitude of recipients and acknowledgments, each individual acknowledgment becomes that much more special to me.

> I have read your poetry and it has
> brought to me such comfort and also
> inspired me to write my feelings down in
> that form. It is a tremendous release.
> I thank you once again for bringing me
> peace through your work.

Although modernity has exiled poetry from the center of society outward to the periphery,[2] I feel that uniting poetry with the now nearly ubiquitous Internet will return the humanities to being on a par with technology. Following is a communication from an Internet correspondent that best illustrates the power of the "new technology" to help lessen the age-old feelings of sorrow:

Dear Dr. Berman,

As I lay in bed this evening waiting, for sleep to come, I realized that I couldn't rest until I wrote to you. Recently I visited your *Hygeia* web site because of a tragedy in my life. I have had three miscarriages in the past year, and I was looking for some hope or comfort through the experiences of others. As I read through your poems, one in particular, "Cameron," seemed so poignant that I copied and saved it. I was moved by it because it reminded me of my best friend's nephew, Alex.

Alex was five years old. He fought a long and difficult battle with leukemia, and then finally a more virulent and pervasive cancer, since his second birthday. He bravely cooperated with his doctors at the hospital. They had tried chemotherapy, a bone marrow transplant, and cord blood transfusion. He had periods of remission and of hope. His parents, devout Catholics, prayed for a miracle, and Alex and his dad even made a pilgrimage to Lourdes, France.

On July 31, Alex's doctors told his parents that he would not live past the weekend. My friend called my husband and me to tell us the sad news. They wanted to organize a tribute to Alex, but were unsure what to do. I discussed it with my husband, a video producer. He immediately suggested a video that would incorporate photographs, music, and video clips of Alex's life. We met with the family on August 1 to assemble the mementos. I remembered your poem and put it in my purse as I was leaving for our meeting.

That evening we chose some music that we all thought was appropriate. But how to end the video? I remembered your poem and suggested it as an end. Everyone loved the poem, and tears flowed as we all read it and realized how appropriate it was. The next day, as my husband started to organize the video, he began with the end, copying your poem in a beautiful script font on a black background. The last two words . . . through Eternity . . . fade into a picture of the Milky Way. The music for the poem is "Friendship Theme" from *Beaches*. We changed one word of the poem, and I am sure you won't mind. We changed the word Nature's to God's, because of the family's deeply religious beliefs.

I just learned that my friend's sweet and brave nephew died today, August 6. I didn't think to write and ask you for approval to use the poem because we were working so quickly, but your name and copyright are included on the cover of the video box, along with the text. The family will be making copies of the video for close relatives.

I would be very honored to send you a copy of the video, if you like. I'm sure that as you watch it, you will be as touched by this little angel and his loving family as all of us have been. And you will also see how appropriate your beautiful poem is.

R. R., Los Gatos, California

The need to reach out to others is both inherent and acquired. There is a "beauty and a tenderness that man can give to man."[3] Through family nurturing and family values, children grow to appreciate that without a thoughtfulness of others, their motives will be selfish and unfulfilling. "No man is an island, entire of itself, every man . . . is a part of the main."[4] We have a need and an obligation to care for others. Physicians, I believe, are in a foremost position to carry out the deeds that they profess through their practice. Whether in academic, research, or clinical practice, laboratory medicine or diagnostic imaging, the physician's role is to bring comfort and to heal others. From such healing come self-reward, self-fulfillment, and honor. If we are surrounded by despair and inequities and have the opportunity to help with their dissolution, it is our obligation to do so. Such is my mission through my work and my poetry. If one person, one family, can be helped or can gather hope through the words I write, it can bring reward equal to that of the healing I perform as a physician. I believe hope is a singular gift we must never destroy. It is an endless song in an endless concert; a nocturne bright in the darkest of nights. Poetry is its instrument, and its music can enable hope.

We as human beings can be distinguished from our ancestors by our capacity to think, to speak, to choose, to consciously procreate, and to understand the value of our actions. To bear children concerns our desire not only to procreate but also to establish a family and instill our values into our offspring. We are not parents without our children, unless our children, conceived through our love and nurtured through our bodies and our spirits, are lost to death. There is such remorse when a child dies or a pregnancy fails: a part of our own humanity is lost, never to be found. Tears cannot adequately portray our grief as we begin a search for reason and comfort. Words we write, words we read, and words we hear can serve as an invaluable source of solace. Words are songs from our hearts and can be "songs of hope, songs for hope."[5]

The Virgin Winter

Let us not succumb to this portent,
The solstice of our darkest hour.
For it is but a finite point
Upon an infinite journey
Which began with all creation and
Upon whose path walk
The souls of our *children*;
Pure as the silence of the virgin winter,
Alive with winds of indomitable hope.

Written in memory of a dear mother and child.

APPENDIX A: A DATABASE OF PERINATAL LOSS

This table represents forty-eight months of registrations to the hygeia.org database and is representative of nearly every type of pregnancy and perinatal loss that can occur. There was a total of 9,023 diagnoses registered of which there was a total of 3,974 known diagnoses (44%). 5,049 (56%) of the registrations were of unknown diagnoses.

Cause of Loss	Number	Percentage
Blighted Ovum/Miscarriage	386	9.70%
Cord Accident	261	6.56%
Incompetant Cervix	253	6.36%
Extreme Prematurity	222	5.58%
Abruptio Placenta	201	5.05%
Chromosomal Trisomy 18	157	3.95%
Ectopic Pregnancy	157	3.95%
Alveolar Capillary Dysplasia	108	2.71%
Premature Rupture of Membranes	107	2.69%
Chromosomal Triplody	87	2.19%
Congenital Heart Disease—Non Specific	84	2.11%
Molar Pregnancy	84	2.11%
Chromosomal Trisomy 21—Down Syndrome	80	2.01%
Anencephaly	77	1.94%
Chorioamnionitis	76	1.91%
Interuterine Fetal Demise—Stillbirth	72	1.81%
Neural Tube Defect	72	1.81%
Asphixia	59	1.48%
Antiphospholipid Antibody Syndrome	56	1.41%
Severe Toxemia	55	1.38%

Multiple Gestation	53	1.33%
Twin to Twin Transfusion Syndrome	52	1.31%
Potter's Syndrome	49	1.23%
Chromosomal Trisomy 13	46	1.16%
Chromosomal Trisomy—Other	37	0.93%
Hypoplastic Left Heart Syndrome	37	0.93%
Sudden Infant Death Syndrome—SIDS	37	0.93%
Turner's Syndrome	37	0.93%
Intrauterine Growth Restriction (IUGR)	35	0.88%
Multiple Congenital Anomalies	30	0.75%
Recurrent Miscarriage	27	0.68%
Group B Strep Chorioamnionitis	25	0.63%
Polycystic Kidney Disease	25	0.63%
Diaphragmatic Hernia	24	0.60%
Diabetes	23	0.58%
Meconium Aspiration Syndrome	21	0.53%
Respiratory Distress Syndrome	19	0.48%
Vanishing Twin Syndrome	19	0.48%
Velamentous Cord Insertion	18	0.45%
Menningitis	16	0.40%
Renal Agenesis	16	0.40%
Hyperemesis—Severe	15	0.38%
True Knot In Cord	15	0.38%
Congenital Anomalies—Non Specific	14	0.35%
Cystic Hygroma	14	0.35%
Lupus Syndrome	14	0.35%
Multiple Losses	14	0.35%
Partial Molar Pregnancy	14	0.35%
Intraventricular Hemorrhage	13	0.33%
Necrotizing Entercolitis	13	0.33%
Chromosomal Abnormality—Not Specified	12	0.30%
Fifth's Disease/Parvo Virus	12	0.30%
Vater Syndrome	12	0.30%
Hydrops Fetalis	11	0.28%
Iatrogenic	11	0.28%
Corpus Luteum Defeciency	10	0.25%
Vasa Previa	10	0.25%
Blood Clot in Cord	9	0.23%
Fibroids/Leiomyomata	9	0.23%
Holoprosencephaly	9	0.23%
Hypoplastic Lung Syndrome	9	0.23%
Loss of One Twin	9	0.23%
Non-Immune Fetal Hydrops	9	0.23%
Omphalocele	9	0.23%
Posterior Urethral Valve Obstruction	8	0.20%
Transposition of Great Vessels	8	0.20%
Twin Pregnancy	8	0.20%
Chromosomal Translocation—Not Specified	7	0.18%

Neonatal Infection	7	0.18%
Chromosomal Trisomy 15	6	0.15%
Chromosomal Trisomy 16	6	0.15%
Fetal Hydrops	6	0.15%
Hormonal Imbalance	6	0.15%
Placental Insufficiency	6	0.15%
Pneumonia	6	0.15%
Staphlococcus Infection	6	0.15%
Bicornuate Uterus	5	0.13%
Blind Tracheal Pouch	5	0.13%
Chromosomal Monosomy	5	0.13%
Genetic Abnormality—Non Specific	5	0.13%
Hypoplastic Left Heart Syndrome	5	0.13%
Hypoxia	5	0.13%
Listeria Infection	5	0.13%
Microcephaly	5	0.13%
Uterine Rupture	5	0.13%
Amniotic Band Syndrome	4	0.10%
Cornual Pregnancy	4	0.10%
Cytomegalovirus (CMV)	4	0.10%
Gastroschesis	4	0.10%
Habitual Abortion	4	0.10%
HELLP Syndrome	4	0.10%
Klinefelter's Syndrome	4	0.10%
LCHAD	4	0.10%
Monoamniotic Twins	4	0.10%
Osteogenesis Imprefecta Type II	4	0.10%
Pseudomonas Pneumonia	4	0.10%
Pulmonary Hypoplasia	4	0.10%
Rh Disease	4	0.10%
Cerebral Dysgenesis	3	0.08%
Chromosomal Ring Chromosome 13	3	0.08%
Chromosomal Trisomy 22	3	0.08%
Chromosomal Trisomy 8	3	0.08%
Chromosomal Trisomy 9	3	0.08%
Congenital Adrenal Hyperplasia	3	0.08%
Cystic Fibrosis	3	0.08%
Double Inlet Left Ventricle	3	0.08%
Endometriosis	3	0.08%
Fetal Distress	3	0.08%
Graves' Disease	3	0.08%
Mitochondrial Depletion Syndrome	3	0.08%
Pneumothorax	3	0.08%
Robert's Syndrome	3	0.08%
Septate Uterus	3	0.08%
Short Rib Polydactyly Syndrome (SRPS)	3	0.08%
Subchorionic Hemorrhage	3	0.08%
Thanatophoric Dysplasia	3	0.08%

Varicella	3	0.08%
Ventriculomegaly	3	0.08%
ACD	2	0.05%
Alobar Holoprosencephaly	2	0.05%
Biliary Atresia	2	0.05%
Bladder Obstruction	2	0.05%
Brain Tumor	2	0.05%
Cardiomyopathy	2	0.05%
Cavernous Hemangioma of the Liver	2	0.05%
Chromosomal Ring Chromosome 21	2	0.05%
Chromosomal Tetraploidy	2	0.05%
Chromosomal Trisomy 14	2	0.05%
Chromosomal Trisomy 14, 15	2	0.05%
Congenital Pneumonia	2	0.05%
Cornelia De Lange	2	0.05%
Dilated Cardiomyopathy	2	0.05%
Dwarfism	2	0.05%
Eclampsia	2	0.05%
Elective Abortion	2	0.05%
Full Term Stillbirth	2	0.05%
Goldenhar Syndrome	2	0.05%
IVF Related	2	0.05%
Luteal Phase Deficinecy	2	0.05%
Maternal Thyroid Disorder	2	0.05%
Oligohydramnios	2	0.05%
Primary Pulmonary Hypertension	2	0.05%
Ruptured Bowel	2	0.05%
Shones Complex	2	0.05%
Shoulder Dystocia	2	0.05%
Smith—Liemli—Optiz	2	0.05%
Suicide Attempt	2	0.05%
Teratoma, Fetal Sacrococcygeal	2	0.05%
Tricuspid Atresia	2	0.05%
Triplet Pregnancy	2	0.05%
Uterine Anomaly	2	0.05%
Volvulous	2	0.05%
Acute Fatty Liver of Pregnancy	1	0.03%
Acute Lactic Acidosis	1	0.03%
Acute Lymphocytic Leukemia—Infant	1	0.03%
Acute Myocardial Infarction	1	0.03%
Adverse Reaction to Necessary Medication	1	0.03%
Age Related Pregnancy Loss	1	0.03%
Agenesis of the Adrenal Gland	1	0.03%
Amniotic Fluid Embolism	1	0.03%
Apnea	1	0.03%
Appendicitis During Pregnancy	1	0.03%
Arrhythmia	1	0.03%
Arthrogryposis	1	0.03%

Atrial Septal Defect	1	0.03%
Autoimmune Problem	1	0.03%
Automobile Accident	1	0.03%
AV Canal	1	0.03%
AVM of the Liver	1	0.03%
Bilateral Pleural Effusions	1	0.03%
Brain Hemorrhage	1	0.03%
Breast and Lung Cancer	1	0.03%
Breast Cancer	1	0.03%
Breech Delivery	1	0.03%
Brown Recluse Spider Bite	1	0.03%
Burn Victim	1	0.03%
Cancer	1	0.03%
Cardiac Arrest of 5½ Week Old	1	0.03%
Cardiac Tamponade	1	0.03%
Cardio Pulminary Stenosis	1	0.03%
Caudal Regression Syndrome	1	0.03%
Cerebal Palsy	1	0.03%
Cerebral Hemorrhage	1	0.03%
Cervical Cancer	1	0.03%
Chemical Pregnancy	1	0.03%
Chromosomal Deletion—Not Specified	1	0.03%
Chromosomal Mosaic Tetrasomy 18p	1	0.03%
Chromosomal Mosaic Trisomy 16	1	0.03%
Chromosomal Translocation, 4–8	1	0.03%
Chromosomal Trisomy 2	1	0.03%
Chromosome Abnormality 4-P	1	0.03%
Chronic Lung Disease	1	0.03%
Clot in Cord	1	0.03%
Congenital Acute Lymphocytic Leukemia	1	0.03%
Congestive Heart Failure	1	0.03%
Corpus Letium Cyst Torsion with Loss of Pregnancy	1	0.03%
Coxsackie Virus	1	0.03%
Crohn's Disease	1	0.03%
Deficiency Of Wharton's Jelly	1	0.03%
DiGeorge Disease With Congential Heart Disease	1	0.03%
Digestive Tract Disorders	1	0.03%
Duodenal Atresia	1	0.03%
Echo 11 Virus	1	0.03%
Ectopia Cordis	1	0.03%
Edwards Syndrome	1	0.03%
Encephalitis	1	0.03%
Encephalocele	1	0.03%
Exomphalus	1	0.03%
Factor V Leiden	1	0.03%
Fetal Alcohol Syndrome	1	0.03%
Fetal Bladder Outlet Obstruction/Prune Belly Syndrome	1	0.03%

Fetal Maternal Hemorrhage	1	0.03%
Fetal Sacrococcygeal Teratoma	1	0.03%
Folic Acid Deficiency	1	0.03%
Gestational Diabetes	1	0.03%
Heart Arrhythmia	1	0.03%
Hemophilia	1	0.03%
Hydranencephaly	1	0.03%
Hydrothorax	1	0.03%
Hypophosphatasia	1	0.03%
Interauterina Hypoxia	1	0.03%
Intrauterine Septum	1	0.03%
Joubert Syndrome	1	0.03%
Limb-Wall Syndrome	1	0.03%
Lissencephaly	1	0.03%
Marfans Syndrome	1	0.03%
Meckel-Gruper Syndrome	1	0.03%
Miscarriage After Amniocentesis	1	0.03%
Miscarriage Due To Physical Abuse	1	0.03%
Missing 1/4 Of 13th Chromosone	1	0.03%
Muscular Dystrophy	1	0.03%
Nager Syndrome	1	0.03%
Niemann-Pick Disease	1	0.03%
Pentology of Cantrell	1	0.03%
Peritonitis Due to Acute Appendicitis	1	0.03%
Poor Egg Response	1	0.03%
Poor Implantation	1	0.03%
Prader-Willi Syndrome, Respiratory Failure	1	0.03%
Pulmonary Stenosis	1	0.03%
Sialidosis	1	0.03%
SLE/Severe Hyperemesis	1	0.03%
Slo-Type II	1	0.03%
Spinal Dysplasia	1	0.03%
Tay Sachs Disease	1	0.03%
Tethered Spine	1	0.03%
Tetralagy of Fallot	1	0.03%
Thrombotic Throbocytopenia Purpuria—TTP	1	0.03%
Torch Syndrome	1	0.03%
Toxoplasmosis	1	0.03%
Tracheal Stenosis	1	0.03%
Trauma	1	0.03%
Tuberous Sclerosis	1	0.03%
Tumor Of The Bladder	1	0.03%
Urea Cycle Defect—Genetic Disorder	1	0.03%
Uterine Bleeding	1	0.03%
Ventricular Septal Defect	1	0.03%
Viral Infection	1	0.03%

Appendix B: Leading Categories of Birth Defects

The estimated incidences for the leading categories of birth defects are provided below. Birth defects are grouped into three major categories: (1) structural/metabolic; (2) congenital infections; and (3) other conditions. Birth defects of the heart and circulatory system affect more infants than any other type. Of all infants born each year, approximately 1 in 115 has heart and/or circulatory defects.

1. Structural/metabolic	Estimated incidence
Heart and circulation	1 in 115 births
Muscles and skeleton	1 in 130 births
Genital/urinary tract	1 in 135 births
Nervous system and eye	1 in 235 births
Chromosomal syndromes	1 in 600 births
Club foot	1 in 735 births
Down syndrome (trisomy 21)	1 in 900 births
Respiratory tract	1 in 900 births
Cleft lip/palate	1 in 930 births
Spina bifida	1 in 2,000 births
Metabolic disorders	1 in 3,500 births
Anencephaly	1 in 8,000 births
PKU	1 in 12,000 births
2. Congenital infection	
Congenital syphilis	1 in 2,000 births
Congenital HIV infection	1 in 2,700 births
Congenital rubella syndrome	1 in 100,000 births

3. Other

Fetal alcohol syndrome	1 in 1,000 births
Rh disease	1 in 1,400 births

Note: All numbers are based on the best available estimates, which underestimate the incidence of many birth defects.

Sources: March of Dimes, Metropolitan Atlanta Congenital Defects Program, and California Birth Defects Monitoring Program.

APPENDIX C: TEN LEADING CAUSES OF INFANT MORTALITY IN THE UNITED STATES IN 1995

Cause of Death	Rate per 100,000 Live Births
Birth defects	168.1
Preterm/low birth weight	100.9
SIDS	87.1
RDS	37.3
Maternal pregnancy complications	33.6
Placental cord compression	24.7
Infections	20.2
Accidents	20.2
Pneumonia/influenza	12.6
Hypoxia/birth asphyxia	12.2

Source: National Center for Health Statistics. Adapted from March of Dimes Perinatal Data Center, 1998.

GLOSSARY

KRISTEN AVERSA, MD

Acute fatty liver of pregnancy. Condition of unknown etiology that occurs most commonly in the third trimester or in the early postpartum period. A patient shows signs and symptoms of liver failure, including nausea, vomiting, increased bleeding time, hematemesis (vomiting blood), and jaundice, as well as abnormal laboratory values signifying liver disease and dysfunction. Treatment is supportive and consists of intravenous fluids, glucose, fresh frozen plasma, and prompt delivery. Mortality has been significantly reduced over the years secondary to early recognition, but there is still a fairly high rate of death. Survivors demonstrate no liver deficits, and there is no increased risk in subsequent pregnancies.

Agenesis of adrenal gland. This congenital lack of the adrenal glands is caused by absence of their progenitor cells during embryogenesis. This extremely rare, but fatal, condition is associated with many other congenital anomalies.

Alveolar capillary dysplasia. A congenital condition in which the capillaries (end unit of the vascular tree) in the lungs of an infant do not make contact with the alveolar (end unit of respiratory tree) epithelium; thus the blood-gas barrier is not formed normally. This is a rare cause of pulmonary hypertension.

Amniotic band syndrome. In utero swallowing, adhering, or constricting of amniotic bands when there is early rupture of the amniotic membrane, causing congenital anomalies including omphalocele, syndactyly (joined fingers or toes), and distorted craniofacial features such as widely separated eyes and displaced nose. The ADAM complex (amniotic deformities, adhesions, mutilation) is a result of this syndrome, but much less severe sequelae may be seen, such as constriction grooves on the limbs. The earlier in gestation the event occurs, the worse the syndrome.

Amniotic fluid embolism. A rare, but most often lethal, event that occurs when a small amount of amniotic fluid enters the vascular system during labor and delivery or placental abruption. The presence of this fluid in the vascular system sets off a cascade of events causing a bleeding problem, vascular collapse, and bronchospasm. Treatment is aimed at supporting the respiratory system and

correcting the shock and coagulopathy. Mechanical ventilation, rapid administration of fluids, and transfusion of blood components should be prompt.

Anencephaly. This is the most severe neural tube defect, the cranial vault is absent or
severely underdeveloped, and the brain is replaced by hemorrhagic tissue. Physical features include a small, thick, and flat skull base.

Antiphospholipid antibody syndrome. An autoimmune disease that in the nonpregnant
state is subclinical but often causes problems during pregnancy from circulating
antibodies that bind to phospholipids. Recurrent abortion, early fetal loss, severe
intrauterine growth retardation, preterm birth, and thromboses are all associated
with this disorder. It usually is not diagnosed until after one of the above events.
Treatment for subsequent pregnancies includes heparin and aspirin.

Asphyxia. A situation in which oxygen supply to the fetus is diminished, causing
hypoxia and acidosis. Causes include placental pathology, acute maternal hypotension, chorioamnionitis, dystocia (difficult labor and delivery), and prolapse,
rupture, or entanglement of the umbilical cord. Any intrapartum death of a
previously healthy fetus should be presumed to be a result of asphyxia until
proven otherwise. Almost every organ system has the potential to become damaged as a result of this condition, including brain tissue (causing neonatal seizures and cerebral palsy). There is an estimated 10% overall mortality rate.

Chorioamnionitis. Inflammation of the chorion and amnion (membranes surrounding
the fetus) secondary to infection. Signs and symptoms include maternal fever
and tachycardia, uterine tenderness, and foul-smelling vaginal discharge. When
bacteria are found in the amniotic fluid, there is an increased incidence of maternal and neonatal sepsis. Premature rupture of membranes increases the likelihood of chorioamnionitis because the bacteria from the lower genital tract
ascend to infect the amniotic cavity. With a positive diagnosis, antibiotics should
be administered promptly and labor should be induced. Prognosis for the neonate is mostly dependent on the gestational age and lung maturity at time of
delivery.

Chromosome deletion. The loss of a portion of DNA, of any length, from a chromosome. Many small deletions are clinically undetectable, while others may
make the difference for different blood groups or for the conditions of cystic
fibrosis or alpha-thalassemia.

Chromosome duplication. A genetic condition in which there is inappropriate duplication of certain areas of DNA on a chromosome. This type of genetic defect
causes certain clinical disorders, including familial hypercholesterolemia.

Chromosome—Klinefelter's syndrome. A syndrome resulting from the trisomy of the
sex chromosomes, in this case 47, XXY. These males are tall and thin, with long
extremities and underdeveloped secondary sexual characteristics. They are always
infertile. A majority of these patients have learning difficulties as well as poor
psychosocial adjustment.

Chromosome marker. Version of a gene that can occupy a particular position on a
chromosome. Markers can be followed through easily classifiable alleles.

Chromosome ring. A rare chromosome that is formed as a result of its ends having
been deleted and the broken arms having united to form a ring.

Chromosome ring 21. A rare chromosomal anomaly that is associated with mental retardation and dysmorphic features. It is rarely familial, but when it is, it is associated with a normal phenotype. In unaffected female carriers, there is an increased risk of having children with Down syndrome.

Chromosome tetraploidy. Condition in which there are four sets of chromosomes instead of two (92, XXXX or 92, XXYY). This condition is incompatible with life, and the fetus is spontaneously aborted early in the pregnancy.

Chromosome translocation. An event that involves the exchange of segments of chromosomes between nonhomologous chromosomes (chromosomes that do not contain the same order of gene positions). A translocation involving chromosome 21 creates the risk of producing a child with Down syndrome.

Chromosome triploidy. A condition that occurs when there are three sets of chromosomes instead of two. The extra set can be paternal (e.g., 69, XXY) or maternal (e.g., 69, XXX). Most abort in the first trimester and may account for up to 10% of all first trimester abortuses. Those which survive into the second trimester may demonstrate intrauterine growth retardation, oligohydramnios (diminished amniotic fluid), facial clefting, abnormalities of the hands and feet, and cranial abnormalities including holoprosencephaly, hydrocephalus, and agenesis of the corpus callosum.

Chromosome trisomy. A state of having three of a given chromosome, instead of the usual pair, that is associated with advanced maternal age. Only three trisomies have been found in postnatal survival (13, 18, 21), and each is associated with growth and mental retardation as well as congenital anomalies.

Chromosome/trisomy 8. This trisomy often demonstrates agenesis of the corpus callosum in the brain (causing holoprosencephaly), cardiac malformations, and facial dysmorphisms. There is also an association with hematological and solid tumors.

Chromosome/trisomy 13. A rare occurrence in live births (it is usually lethal by six months). Clinical characteristics include growth retardation, central nervous system malformations including holoprosencephaly, severe mental retardation, absence of the eyes, cleft lip and palate, polydactyly, rocker-bottom feet, and congenital heart and urogenital defects. Advanced maternal age is a risk factor.

Chromosome/trisomy 14. A rare trisomy that is associated with malignancy.

Chromosome/trisomy 15. A rare trisomy, usually aborted in the first trimester. In live births, its severity depends on the degree of mosaicism, such as dysmorphism of the nose, anomalies of the hands and feet, and hematological malignancies.

Chromosome/trisomy 16. The most common trisomy in abortuses; it is not seen in live births.

Chromosome/trisomy 18. A rare condition in live-born infants; it is estimated that about 95% of fetuses with this chromosomal abnormality abort spontaneously. Postnatal survival is usually only a few months. Features of this condition include mental retardation, failure to thrive, and severe congenital malformations of the heart. Ears are low-set, feet are rocker-bottom, the jaw is receding, and the fists are clenched (the second and fifth digits overlap the third and fourth). As with most trisomies, advanced maternal age is a risk factor.

Chromosome/trisomy 21 (Down syndrome). The most common chromosomal disorder, occurring in about 1 in 800 live births, with an elevated risk occurring in
children or fetuses of mothers older than thirty-five. Clinical features include
characteristic eyes, short stature, flat nasal bridge, low-set ears, protruding
tongue, single crease in palm ("simian crease"), a wide gap between the first and
second toes, and mental retardation. Congenital heart disease is very common,
as are gastrointestinal anomalies (duodenal atresia and tracheoesophageal fistula),
and there is a steep increase in the risk of leukemia. About half of these patients
survive beyond fifty years, and there is a premature senility similar to Alzheimer's
disease that occurs in a large percentage of people with Down syndrome. This
disease, well known to be associated with advanced maternal age, can be
screened for by the triple screen test (low alpha-fetoprotein, low unconjugated
estriol, and elevated human chorionic gonadotropin) and later confirmed by
diagnostic amniocentesis with chromosomal analysis.

Chromosome/trisomy 22. The most frequent trisomy, after trisomy 16, in spontaneous
abortions. Patients with this trisomy can survive if it is expressed in its mosaic
form, but they always have many physical anomalies, including microcephaly,
heart defects, craniofacial dysmorphisms, hypoplasia of the fingers, and mental
retardation. This chromosomal event is associated with advanced maternal age.

Chromosome—Turner's syndrome. Found in females with the karyotype 45, X instead
of 46, XX, resulting in a syndrome that includes short stature, gonadal dysgenesis
(streak ovaries), infertility, unusual facies, webbing of the neck, widely spaced
nipples, increased risk of cardiovascular and renal anomalies, and a deficiency in
spatial abilities and motor organization. Intelligence is usually normal. There is
a very high incidence of this chromosomal abnormality in spontaneous abortions,
but it seems to be very compatible with postnatal survival.

CMV. This is a DNA virus that can be transmitted through blood transfusion, organ
transplant, sexual contact, transplacentally, during delivery, as well as through
breast-feeding, saliva, and urine. Over half of pregnant women demonstrate ser-
opositivity for CMV, indicating that they have been infected and that the virus
could be in latency. Subclinical infection is the usual course, though, a mono-
like illness may ensue. During pregnancy, a fetus may become infected even
when the mother is asymptomatic, with 10%–20% of the neonates exhibiting a
congenital syndrome including nonimmune hydrops, intrauterine growth retardation, chorioretinitis, microcephaly, cerebral calcifications, hydrocephaly, and
enlargement of the liver and spleen. The severity of this syndrome is not dependent on when in the pregnancy a woman incurred the infection, and there
is a much lower fetal risk when the infection in the mother is a recurrent one.
Many infants are asymptomatic at birth but later develop mental retardation,
psychomotor delay, and progressive hearing loss. There is no treatment for this
virus, but ultrasound and amniotic fluid culture can help to diagnose fetal infection.

Congenital adrenal hyperplasia. An autosomal recessive disorder (requiring inheritance of two genes to manifest disease) in which an enzyme deficiency in the
adrenal gland (most often 21-hydroxylase) causes virilization of females secondary to the overproduction of androgenic hormones. In utero exposure of the

female fetus to high levels of these adrenal androgens results in an infant with ambiguous genitalia, though the ovaries, fallopian tubes, and uterus are unaffected. A male infant usually appears normal at birth. In about half of affected individuals, there is also life-threatening salt wasting. Treatment is both medical and surgical, including administration of glucocorticoids and correction of the ambiguous genitalia.

Congenital heart disease. Cardiovascular malformations that occur in approximately 1% of all live births. The etiology is unclear; only 5%–10% can be explained by maternal infection, toxic exposure, or chromosomal abnormalities. There are many different forms that this condition can take, including malformations of the great arteries, heart valves, outflow tracts (aorta and pulmonary arteries), and septa (walls between the chambers of the heart). Many fetuses with severe cardiac defects die in utero. Treatment for an affected infant depends on the type of defect and usually includes surgery: grafts, flaps, shunts, and even heart transplant.

Cord accident. An event such as prolapse or rupture of the umbilical cord that causes the temporary or permanent disruption of blood flow to the fetus prior to birth or during delivery. This is a grave situation because the flow of oxygenated blood is blocked from the fetus. Prolapse of the cord may occur with excessively long cords or with malpresentation of the fetus during delivery. Rupture of a short cord may cause acute fetal blood loss. Fetal monitoring helps to initiate prompt management.

Diabetes. Glucose intolerance caused by autoimmune pancreatic dysfunction with low/absent production of insulin (type I) or by tissue resistance to insulin (type II), both causing hyperglycemia. These may be present prior to pregnancy or may be caused or unveiled during pregnancy. Prior or "overt" diabetes carries with it greater morbidity and mortality for the mother and fetus than does "gestational" diabetes, and used to be the cause of much infertility. Depending on the degree of glycemic control at conception and during early embryogenesis, there is still a risk for spontaneous abortion. Half of spontaneous abortions are associated with fetal anomalies, intrauterine fetal demise, intrauterine growth retardation, congenital anomalies including cardiovascular or neural tube defects, caudal regression syndrome, macrosomia (fetus weighing more than 4000 g) with traumatic delivery, and delayed organ maturity. There is an increased risk for neonatal hypoglycemia within minutes of birth, due to an overstimulated fetal pancreas as a result of in utero exposure to maternal hyperglycemia. For the mother, there is an increased risk of polyhydramnios, preeclampsia, ketoacidosis, and infection. Overt diabetes during pregnancy may or may not have an adverse effect on retinopathy, neuropathy, or nephropathy established from the preexisting diabetes. Gestational diabetes develops as an overresponse to normal insulin resistance during pregnancy with hyperglycemia. It has a greater incidence in obese women and typically occurs later in gestation. Interestingly, over half of these women will develop overt diabetes later in life, and there is the possibility that their offspring have increased risk for obesity and diabetes as well. There is not the same risk for fetal anomalies as there is with overt diabetes, since the hyperglycemia does not usually occur during embryogenesis. However, there is still the risk of having a macrosomic infant, which increases the risk of morbidity and mortality secondary to shoulder dystocia. Gestational diabetes also carries the risk for neonatal hypoglycemia, as well as for unexplained stillbirth. Detection of diabetes during pregnancy is first done by the one-hour glucose tolerance test, followed by the three-hour glucose tolerance test for borderline one-hour tests. Treatment is through diet, exercise, and insulin as hyperglycemia increases as the gestation progresses. There is a very high recurrence for subsequent pregnancies.

Diaphragmatic hernia. A condition that may occur in utero in the developing fetus when part or all of its bowel enters the thoracic (chest) cavity through an enlarged hole in the diaphragm. The bowel contents take up space, thus inhibiting growth of the lungs, which results in pulmonary hypoplasia and pulmonary hypertension, both of which cause neonatal cyanosis. This disorder manifests a scaphoid (sunken) abdomen, respiratory distress, and bowel sounds in the chest on auscultation. Treatment is respiratory support and surgery.

DiGeorge's syndrome. A disease that is caused by congenital absence of the parathyroid and thymus glands due to abnormal development early in organogenesis. It is classified as a sporadic syndrome complex of unknown etiology and is associated with micrognathia (underdeveloped jaw), as well as aortic arch anomalies. The disease may present with hypocalcemia secondary to absence of parathyroid hormone, as well as increased susceptibility to infection from diminished T-cell production due to lack of the thymus gland.

Dilated cardiomyopathy. Often called congestive cardiomyopathy, this disorder can be categorized into three groups: myocarditis, primary (familial), and drug-induced. Myocarditis is related to viral infections such as the Coxsackie virus and is usually diagnosed during an episode of heart failure. An echocardiogram shows a very large and dilated heart. Patients are given diuretics and digitalis, and usually recover completely.

Eclampsia. This is preeclampsia with the addition of grand mal seizures. Patients with severe preeclampsia are at greater risk, but eclampsia does occur in mild forms as well. Management includes oxygen, intravenous fluids with dextrose, antihypertensive drugs (hydralazine), magnesium sulfate to decrease the hyperreflexia and prevent further convulsions, and delivery.

Ectopic pregnancy. A gestation that implants outside of the endometrial cavity, most often in the fallopian tubes, causing a serious hazard to the woman's health. Risk factors identified include prior or current history of pelvic inflammatory disease (PID), history of therapeutic abortion, tubal ligation, prior ectopic pregnancy, intrauterine device (IUD), and DES exposure. The overall incidence is high, occurring in approximately 1 in 200 pregnancies. Symptoms of the condition include amenorrhea, vaginal bleeding, abdominal pain, referred shoulder pain, and, if ruptured, often a shocklike picture. Diagnosis is initiated by maternal blood test for levels of beta-HCG abnormal for those of an intrauterine pregnancy. Ultrasound is next employed to identify the location of the sac, and surgical laparoscopy or laparotomy is performed to remove the gestation. Drugs (methotrexate) have gained popularity and may be infused intravenously for several days or directly into the gestational sac.

Extreme prematurity. Preterm infants have much more morbidity and mortality than full-term infants, due to their underdevelopment. Because not all of the maternal antibodies that provide immunity for the infant have crossed the placenta, neonates born before 32 weeks are at a sixfold greater risk of becoming septic. These infants also usually cannot coordinate the mechanisms for oral feeding, so they need to be fed through a nasal or oral gastric tube. Immaturity of the gastrointestinal tract may precipitate gastroesophageal reflux, gastric stasis, abdominal distention and obstruction, inability to defecate, reflux and aspiration, as well as intolerance to certain elements of milk. Extremely early newborns, especially those weighing under 750g, are also at increased risk for neonatal hypoglycemia, retinopathy and blindness, hearing loss, hydrocephalus, microcephaly, mental retardation, cerebral palsy, chronic pulmonary insufficiency, necrotizing enterocolitis with subsequent short bowel syndrome, intraventricular hemorrhage and seizures, growth failure, and learning disabilities.

Factor V leiden (activated protein C resistance). This is an inherited state of hypercoagulability in which one is prone to venous thrombosis (clotting). In pregnancy, it is the cause of recurrent abortions, and it is thought to be associated with the development of preeclampsia.

Fetal demise (intrauterine fetal death IUFD). Death of the fetus after 20 weeks' gestation but before onset of labor. The estimated occurrence is approximately 1% of all pregnancies, with about half having an unknown etiology. Identified causes include placental and cord complications, maternal hypertension or medical condition, congenital anomalies of the fetus, and intrauterine infection. Signs include absence of fetal movement, uterus small for dates, absence of fetal heart tones, but not necessarily a negative pregnancy test (the placenta may continue to produce beta-HCG). Definitive diagnosis is made by ultrasound. Approaches to management usually include induction of labor to ease the emotional component of the loss as well as to reduce the chance of intrauterine infection or disseminated intravascular coagulation and shock. However, most women go into spontaneous labor within a couple of weeks. If etiology is not apparent, further investigation should follow, including maternal blood tests, fetal chromosomal studies, and bacterial and viral cultures.

Fetal distress. A condition that occurs when a fetus is unable to maintain biochemical homeostasis and becomes acidotic and hypoxic as a result of intrapartum asphyxia. Causes include problems with the umbilical cord (vasa previa, nuchal cord, prolapse), placenta (infarction, abruption), fetus (anemia, infection) or mother (hypertension or hypotension, anemia, heart disease, seizure activity, pulmonary disease). This condition is screened by electronic fetal monitor demonstrating abnormal heart rate patterns. Management is dependent on the cause, but change of maternal position, oxygen therapy, and close monitoring of maternal and fetal conditions are routinely employed.

Fetal hydrops. See Hydrops fetalis, immune.

Fetal-maternal hemorrhage. The presence of fetal red blood cells in the maternal circulation, which can be identified by a specific test (Kleihauer-Betke) that detects fetal hemoglobin. With this test and the mother's hematocrit, the amount of fetal blood loss can be calculated. Large bleeds are uncommon and are associated with a placental lesion such as a chorioangioma. If there is a placental abruption due to trauma, there is an increased risk of this type of hemorrhage.

Fetal sacrococcygeal teratoma. A teratoma is a tumor arising from several different cell lines and contains many types of tissue. A sacrococcygeal teratoma is the most common teratoma in newborns and occurs in females more than males. It may be very large but can be fully removed through surgery, which should be performed on the first day of life in order to reduce the chance of development into malignancy. Diagnosis is by ultrasound, and complications include dystocia (difficult birth), nonimmune hydrops, polyhydramnios (excess amniotic fluid), and bleeding from tears. It is not typically accompanied by other anomalies.

Goldenhar syndrome. A syndrome of malformations including the face, tongue, soft palate, and ears that may or may not have an associated deafness. It is caused by disruption early in embryogenesis, of unknown etiology.

Graves' disease. An autoimmune disease caused by receptor antibodies causing hyperthyroidism. In pregnancy these antibodies can cross the placenta, with the potential to cause neonatal thyrotoxicosis in 1% of newborns born to women with Graves' disease. This is usually a transient state, but it carries a significant risk of mortality. Intrapartum, the fetus may demonstrate growth retardation. The disease actually improves for the woman during pregnancy but may exacerbate in the postpartum period. Labor, infection, cesarean section, or noncompliance with medications may precipitate "thyroid storm" or intense thyrotoxicosis with a 25% rate of maternal mortality. New-onset Graves' disease is difficult to diagnose during pregnancy, because signs and symptoms of hyperthyroidism include those seen in the hyperdynamic circulatory state of a normal pregnancy. Total serum levels of thyroid hormones (specifically T4) are measured to make the diagnosis. Treatment during pregnancy is a bit different—radioactive iodine is contraindicated, but the other medical (PTU [Propylthiouracil] or Tapazole) or surgical options are utilized. PTU, however, does cross the placenta and carries a 1%–5% risk of creating fetal goiter and hypothyroidism.

Group B Strep (GBS). A type of streptococcal bacteria that is part of the normal gastrointestinal flora of humans and can be found in the vagina, cervix, throat, skin, and urethra. If a woman carries GBS in her vagina during pregnancy, there may be transmission to the infant at delivery. Other risk factors for transmission include preterm labor and delivery, prolonged labor, preterm rupture of membranes, intrapartum fever, and a low birth weight infant. This organism is the most common cause of neonatal sepsis in the United States. The infection can be divided into early onset and late onset; early onset usually presents within forty-eight hours as respiratory distress, pneumonia, and often meningitis secondary to vertical transmission. Antibiotics must be initiated immediately. Despite expedient efforts, there is a very high mortality, especially in preterm infants. Late onset is usually acquired in the neonatal nursery and presents by four weeks of life, most often as meningitis. Effective measures to decrease this life-threatening infection for infants are mass screening of pregnant women and initiation of antibiotics during labor; antibiotic administration prior to labor and delivery has not been shown to prevent transmission.

HELLP syndrome. An acronym that stands for hemolysis, elevated liver enzymes, and low platelets. The syndrome is an uncommon variant of preeclampsia, differing in that it occurs more often in multiparous (having had more than one baby) women, women over twenty-five years old, and gestations less than 36 weeks. Hypertension may be absent. Diagnosis is made by clinical signs as well as maternal blood tests. Management of this condition includes delivery if the pregnancy is more than 34 weeks or there is evidence of fetal lung maturity in combination with signs of deteriorating health of either the mother or the fetus. Elements of this syndrome usually correct themselves shortly after delivery, but usually the coagulopathy is stabilized and supportive measures are provided.

Holoprosencephaly. A condition in which there is a single undivided hemisphere in the brain rather than the normal two hemispheres. This is due to agenesis of the corpus callosum in the brain, and it is often accompanied by facial dysmorphology including cyclopia, hypoplastic eyes, agnathia, otocephaly, and facial clefts. Many fetuses with this condition also have a chromosomal disturbance, most often trisomy 13 or 18.

Hydrocephaly. A condition in which there is an enlargement of the ventricles in the brain that house the cerebrospinal fluid (CSF). The etiology is through obstruction of CSF along its course, often as a result of congenital malformations of the brain, brain stem, or bones of the skull. Increased intracranial pressure is a manifestation of this condition, which eventually causes neurological problems such as ataxia, spasticity, atrophy of the optic nerve, and endocrine dysfunction. Treatment is both medical and surgical, including drugs that decrease the production of CSF and shunts that bypass the obstructive site.

Hydrops fetalis. Abnormal accumulation of fluid in the tissue (edema/anasarca) and body cavities (pericardial/pleural effusions and ascites) of the fetus as well as excess amniotic fluid (polyhydramnios). Diagnosis is made by a thorough history from the mother that covers race, occupation, infectious exposures, and obstetrical, medical, and family history. Blood work should entail a complete blood count, chemistry, protein, genetics, and viral and bacterial cultures. A comprehensive ultrasound should also be performed to assess the fetus's anatomy and well-being. This condition is treated according to the etiology. When associated with structural heart disease, it is almost always fatal. In addition to fetal loss, other severe sequelae include prematurity secondary to polyhydramnios and bilateral pulmonary hypoplasia as a result of growth interference by the fluid that occupied the pleural cavity during development. Maternal complications include hypoproteinemia, edema, hypertension, pregnancy-induced hypertension, and uterine overdistension secondary to polyhydramnios, with the associated dangers of abruption, cord prolapse, and postpartum hemorrhage.

Hydrops-Immune. Hydrops caused by maternal circulating antibodies acting against the fetal red blood cells, resulting in anemia of the fetus with subsequent tissue hypoxia and heart failure. The antibodies are formed in response to maternal exposure to fetal blood cells in a prior pregnancy, delivery, or abortion. The most common antibody is to the Rh antigen on the fetal cells, and the immune response (and thus the hydrops) can be prevented by administration of Rh immune globulin at 28 weeks and in the immediate postpartum period. Treatment of this form of hydrops includes in utero fetal transfusion.

Hydrops-Nonimmune. Uncommon during a viable pregnancy but found commonly in first and second trimester spontaneous abortions. The many causes of this condition can be separated into fetal, maternal, and placental etiologies. Fetal causes include anatomic anomalies (cardiovascular, thoracic, gastrointestinal, urinary tract), chromosomal abnormalities (45X; trisomy 13, 18, and 21), infection (CMV, parvovirus B19, toxoplasmosis, syphilis, Coxsackie, rubella, *Listeria*), anemia (secondary to alpha-thalassemia, G6PD deficiency, maternal-fetal hemorrhage, twin-to-twin transfusion), or metabolic disorders. Maternal causes include severe diabetes mellitus, anemia, or hypoproteinemia. Placental causes include chorioangioma, venous thrombosis, and cord torsion or knot.

Hyperemesis gravidarum. A condition defined by intractable nausea and vomiting that has an estimated incidence of 1% of all pregnancies. It occurs most frequently in white women in a first pregnancy. Diagnosis is by history and physical exam. The illness is self-limiting and the outcome is generally good, though it may be complicated by metabolic deterioration as a result of dehydration and electrolyte loss. Treatment includes psychosocial support and counseling, dietary modifications, and antiemetic drugs when other approaches have failed.

Hypoplastic left heart syndrome. A syndrome that includes the in utero underdevelopment of the left ventricular chamber in the heart (which pumps oxygenated blood to the brain and body). Fetuses with these congenital anomalies do well in utero, but post parturition their condition quickly declines, demonstrating heart failure, low cardiac output, cyanosis, and acidosis. Treatment requires surgery; otherwise early neonatal death will ensue. Options include a two-step operation (the second at about two years of age) or a cardiac transplant.

Hypoplastic lung syndrome (pulmonary hypoplasia). A congenital disorder that ultimately causes pulmonary hypertension and pulmonary insufficiency and presents as respiratory distress in the neonate. This condition may be due to decreased amniotic fluid (a substance that is needed to prevent constriction of the fetus by the uterus), which inhibits lung growth; any bone disorders, where the chest wall is small and bony, prevent proper development; diaphragmatic hernias and pleural effusions in hydrops fetalis, which act as space-occupying lesions in the chest cavity, thus inhibiting appropriate development of the lungs; and neuromuscular diseases that prevent normal fetal breathing movement, which is needed for lung growth and maturation. Treatment includes admission to the Neonatal Intensive Care Unit, intubation, and treatment with steroids and surfactant.

Incompetent cervix. A condition in which the cervix is unable to hold a pregnancy because it prematurely dilates. Causes are anatomical, usually secondary to trauma from a rapid dilation during a pregnancy termination or curettage, as well as functional (the cervix is anatomically indistinguishable from a normal cervix yet is associated with pregnancy loss). In subsequent pregnancies, a suture or cerclage is placed through the cervix in the first trimester to prevent premature dilation and pregnancy loss.

Intrauterine growth retardation (IUGR). A condition defined by a neonatal birth weight less than the tenth percentile for any given gestational age. Risk factors include previous low birth weight infants; short maternal stature and weight less than 100 pounds; narcotic, alcohol, and cigarette use; chronic hypertension;

pregnancy-induced hypertension; threatened abortion; intrauterine infection; and congenital malformation of the fetus. The fetus is at risk for meconium aspiration, asphyxia, hypoglycemia, and mental retardation. Diagnosis, made by ultrasound, includes precise measurements of fetal head and abdominal circumference, femur length, and estimated fetal weight (all dependent on accurate dating). Intrapartum management consists of bed rest and correction of underlying cause. Prognosis is good if there is no underlying chromosomal disruption, congenital anomaly, or infection, but a neonatal team must be on hand because the neonate is at risk for hypoglycemia, hypothermia, and respiratory distress.

Intraventricular hemorrhage. A condition usually occurring in the first three days of life that is more prevalent in preterm and very low birth weight infants and is a common cause of neonatal seizures. The pathogenesis of the bleeding is unknown, although there are many theories, such as weak blood vessels and unstable blood pressure of the neonate. Diagnosis is confirmed by ultrasound through the anterior fontanelle, and treatment includes supportive care, blood transfusions, and shunts to decrease the intracranial pressure.

LCHAD. A defect in mitochondrial fatty acid oxidation involving the enzyme 3-hydroxyacyl-CoA dehydrogenase. In the pregnant woman with this disease or who is a carrier of this gene, there is an increased risk of severe preeclampsia or acute fatty liver changes of pregnancy. In the neonate, this disease manifests as hypoglycemia, hepatopathy, hypotonia, cardiomyopathy, retinopathy, and hypoparathyroidism. Treatment is dietary modification.

Listeria. A bacterium that occurs in unpasteurized milk and is found in chickens, pigs, and even in the fecal flora of humans. It may cause listeriosis, a very rare illness that is usually mild and self-limiting during pregnancy. However, it may cause preterm labor or chorioamnionitis. Transplacental infection may result in spontaneous abortion, intrauterine fetal demise, and sepsis, meningitis, conjunctivitis, and respiratory infection in the newborn, as well as neonatal death. An infected placenta demonstrates characteristic small areas of necrosis and abscesses. Ampicillin and gentamicin can be administered during pregnancy.

Luteal phase defect. The luteal phase begins with the onset of the luteinizing hormone midcycle surge that initiates ovulation and ends with the first day of menses. It is concurrent with the secretory phase of the endometrium (dynamic lining of the uterine cavity), which is when this lining prepares itself for implantation of a fertilized egg. Progesterone is the hormone that dominates these two periods. A defect during the luteal phase is a cause of infertility that may be suggested by an abnormal increase in basal body temperature, a history of spontaneous abortion, or demonstration of poor cervical mucus. Endometrial biopsy with careful histologic examination, providing the exact dating of the menstrual cycle is known, can make the diagnosis.

Meconium aspiration syndrome. A syndrome that usually occurs in full-term infants. It causes neonatal cyanosis and respiratory distress through mechanical obstruction, inflammation from chemical pneumonitis, and pulmonary hypertension. Meconium in the amniotic fluid signifies fetal distress, and it is common in infants born in the breech presentation. Aspiration of this fluid can happen in utero, but more commonly occurs immediately after delivery. Many of these infants develop pneumonia or pneumothorax. Treatment is supportive care as well as mechanical ventilation. Prevention is through careful fetal monitoring, close observation of the fluid that comes out during birth, and immediate suctioning of the oropharynx before delivering the infant's body. After full delivery, deeper and more aggressive suctioning should be instituted. Some doctors practice saline infusion into the amniotic cavity prior to delivery, in the belief that this may reduce the incidence of aspiration.

Meningitis. This is the inflammation of the tissue layer that surrounds the brain and spinal cord; it may be caused by bacteria, viruses, or (uncommonly) fungi. The three most common bacterial organisms that cause meningitis in the neonatal period are group B strep, *Listeria monocytogenes* and *E. coli*, which usually result from late-onset sepsis. Despite antibiotics, there is still a high mortality for infants with meningitis, especially if born preterm. Among the survivors of bacterial meningitis, there is a high incidence of neurological abnormalities. The most common viruses causing neonatal meningitis are rubella, CMV, herpes, Coxsackie and echo virus, typically from intrauterine transplacental infection.

Microcephaly. "Small head," one that is more than three standard deviations below the mean size, due to any process that causes brain growth to stop in the perinatal period. Etiologies include chromosomal, genetic, infectious (congenital rubella, CMV, *Herpes simplex*, toxoplasmosis, and syphilis), toxic (maternal radiation or alcohol), or vascular (intrauterine or neonatal hypoxia/ischemia). One treatable cause of this disorder is premature closure of the skull sutures associated with hyperthyroidism. Microcephalic children are usually free of other anomalies but do have impaired intellectual development.

Miscarriage. This is the lay term for a spontaneous event that ends a pregnancy. This event is called "abortion" in medical terminology and is defined as the unplanned, spontaneous loss of a pregnancy before the fetus can survive outside the mother or if the fetus is less than 500g or 20 weeks' gestation. There are several types of abortion: threatened, inevitable, incomplete, complete, missed, and recurrent. Threatened abortion is a pregnancy that is complicated by vaginal bleeding before 20 weeks' gestation with a closed cervix. Approximately 25% of pregnancies are threatened abortions, and 50% of these go on to abort completely. An inevitable abortion is a pregnancy complicated by vaginal bleeding, cramping and dilation. The pregnancy is eventually lost. An incomplete abortion consists of vaginal bleeding, dilation, and passage of some products of conception. A complete abortion is defined by passage of all products of conception, decreased uterine contractions, closed cervix, and a negative pregnancy test. A missed abortion occurs when a fetus has died but is retained in the uterus for some weeks. Recurrent abortion is defined as three successive abortions, although most clinicians consider two successive first trimester or one second trimester loss reason for investigation. Blighted ovum is an abortion where there is no visible fetus in the sac.

Molar pregnancy. "Gestational trophoblastic neoplasia" (GTN) is a condition that comes in several forms which vary in levels of severity: benign hydatidiform mole (subdivided into complete and partial, according to genetic makeup), invasive mole, and malignant choriocarcinoma. The cause of molar pregnancy is un-

GLOSSARY

known, and the pathophysiology is defective fertilization. Incidence in the Far East is much greater than in the United States. Risk of a second molar pregnancy is approximately forty times greater after the first. Symptoms of a molar pregnancy include a uterus large for dates, irregular/heavy bleeding, hyperthyroid-type symptoms, occasional hyperemesis gravidarum, or preeclampsia. Diagnosis is by high levels of beta-HCG, confirmed by an ultrasound that shows a "snow storm" appearance. In benign hydatidiform moles, the complete mole is comprised of an empty egg (no maternal genetic material) that was fertilized, and thus contains only paternal chromosomes; partial moles consist of an egg with genetic material fertilized by two sperm. A partial mole is associated with a developing fetus, symptoms are usually less severe, and there is a lower malignant potential. Invasive moles demonstrate persistent beta-HCG despite molar evacuation. They rarely metastasize, so hysterectomy is usually curative. Half of malignant choriocarcinomas follow a molar pregnancy, and the other half precede a spontaneous or induced abortion or an ectopic pregnancy. Symptoms mimic many other diseases and malignancies, so unless choriocarcinoma follows a molar pregnancy, it is usually not suspected. Malignant choriocarcinoma metastasizes and is treated with chemotherapy (radiation therapy if it metastasizes to the brain or liver). This disease is divided into good and bad prognostic features (such as metastases to the brain or liver, very high beta-HCG titres, occurrence after a full-term delivery) predicting chance of survival. Cure is possible in most instances of cases with good prognostic features.

Monoamniotic twins. Twins that share an amniotic cavity without membranes to separate them. They may also share a chorion (monochorionic), with the possibility of having two umbilical cords or sharing one cord that is forked. In the monoamniotic condition there was very late cleavage (splitting) of the fertilized egg. The later the cleavage, the more parts will be shared by the embryos, including body parts that produce "conjoined twins." This type of pregnancy has the risks of any multiple pregnancy, including intrauterine growth retardation, preterm birth, congenital anomalies, and velamentous insertion of the cord, but it carries the additional risk of cord entanglement because there are no membranes between the fetuses.

Multicystic (polycystic) kidneys. This is an inherited disease that affects both kidneys and comes in two forms: autosomal recessive (requires inheritance of two genes for expression), referred to as "infantile," and autosomal dominant (requiring only one gene for expression), referred to as "adult" polycystic kidney disease. The infantile form is characterized by enlargement of the kidneys as a result of the many cysts throughout. This can be diagnosed in utero by ultrasound. Due to oligohydramnios (too little amniotic fluid) from poorly functioning fetal kidneys, pulmonary hypoplasia occurs because the lungs need this fluid to develop properly. This is the cause of much of the morbidity and mortality. Hepatic (liver) fibrosis also occurs with this form of the disease and contributes to the high degree of morbidity and mortality. The adult type typically occurs in the fourth or fifth decade of life, but can present in early childhood or even infancy. This form is associated with a strong family history; hepatic, splenic, and pancreatic cysts; and cerebral aneurysms.

Multiple gestation. Defined as any pregnancy in which there is more than one embryo or fetus. This is considered a complication of pregnancy because it has a much higher morbidity and mortality for the fetuses as well as for the mother. The etiology of this phenomenon is through the splitting of fertilized egg or through the fertilization of more than one egg, the first being termed monozygotic (identical) and the second being dizygotic (fraternal). Dizygotic fetuses have separate fetal membranes (chorion and amnion), but the placentas may be separate or fused. Monozygotic fetuses may be the result of cleavage of the egg at several stages during early embryogenesis; the later the cleavage occurs, the more parts of the membranes, cord, or even the fetuses are shared. Monozygosity also creates the risk of twin-twin transfusion, placental vascular anastomosis (connections between the arterial and venous circulation), and fetal or umbilical cord malformations. Both types of multiple gestation are associated with preterm labor and delivery, and all of the morbidity and mortality accompanying these processes. There are also maternal complications of multiple gestations, such as anemia, hypertension, postpartum uterine atony, postpartum hemorrhage, and preeclampsia and eclampsia. The prevalence of multiple gestation varies according to race, heredity, maternal age, and the use of fertility agents (10%–30% of pregnancies are multiple, depending on the type of therapy used). Diagnosis is confirmed through ultrasound, but signs and symptoms include excessive maternal weight gain and fetal movement, and more than one fetal heartbeat found during auscultation. Management includes measures that will prolong the gestation, such as bed rest and tocolytic therapy to prevent preterm labor, close fetal monitoring by ultrasound, and steroids to increase fetal lung maturity if preterm labor ensues. The mode of delivery is dependent on the presentation of the fetuses.

Necrotizing enterocolitis. A medical emergency that usually occurs in the premature infant who is receiving oral feedings. Symptoms usually begin in the first week of life and include abdominal tenderness and distention, rectal bleeding, and a shocklike appearance; positive blood cultures occur in less than half of the patients. Diagnosis is by X-ray, and treatment includes antibiotics, nasogastric decompression, and parenteral (through the veins) nutrition. A grave consequence is intestinal perforation, which requires surgical exploration.

Neonatal sepsis. This is a severe systemic illness of the newborn that can be acquired in utero or during delivery. It presents as early or late onset, or can be acquired after birth, in the nursery. Important organisms include group B strep, *Staphylococcus aureus* and *epidermidis*, and *Listeria*. Early onset sepsis from in utero exposure usually occurs in premature infants and presents as grunting, tachypnea, and cyanosis at birth. The disease manifests as respiratory failure, shock, meningitis, necrosis of the functional units of the kidneys, peripheral gangrene, hypoxia, and hypotension. Risk factors include vaginal colonization with the causative organism (e.g., group B strep), preterm or prolonged rupture of membranes, chorioamnionitis, male sex, black race, and preterm birth. Treatment includes antibiotics, mechanical ventilation, and medication to keep the blood pressure up. Late onset neonatal sepsis occurs after the first week of life, usually in a healthy full-term infant. This variation presents as lethargy, poor feeding, hypotonia, apathy, seizures, bulging fontanelles, fever, and bacteremia; it may result in focal infection (such as urinary tract infection or osteomyelitis) from seeding through the blood. Treatment is the same as for early onset. Acquired sepsis usually occurs in preterm infants who are exposed to pathogens, typically multidrug-resistant organisms, in the Neonatal Intensive Care Unit, because these infants often have indwelling catheters, endotracheal tubes, and central venous lines, which are excellent conduits for infection. Sepsis in these infants can present in many ways, including pneumonia, meningitis, cellulitis, and diarrhea. Treatment is with antibiotics effective against resistant organisms.

Neural tube defect. One of the most common malformation; it may include the cranium and/or the spinal cord. There is a wide range in severity, from lethal (anencephaly) to asymptomatic (spina bifida occulta). It is diagnosed by measuring the amniotic fluid level of alpha-fetoprotein, as well as a through a comprehensive ultrasound after 16 weeks' gestation. Etiologies of this group of defects include teratogens, single gene mutations, and chromosomal abnormalities.

Niemann-Pick disease. This disease is one of the lysosomal storage diseases caused by deficiency of the enzyme sphingomyelin. It is autosomal recessive, requiring inheritance of two genes to manifest the disease. Presentation may occur in utero, as hydrops fetalis, or late in adulthood. Manifestations include intellectual retardation, seizures, loss of muscle tone, enlargement of the liver and spleen, and jaundice. Diagnosis can be confirmed by enzyme analysis of blood leukocytes (white blood cells) or skin fibroblast, by investigation of bone marrow, and by chorionic villus sampling in the first trimester of pregnancy.

Omphalocele. Herniation of abdominal contents into the umbilical cord caused by a midline ventral defect. This condition is associated with other major malformations (cardiac, gastrointestinal, genitourinary, musculoskeletal, central nervous system) as well as with chromosomal disruptions. The associated condition determines the prognosis, but there is approximately 90% survival if the omphalocele is isolated. Incidence is probably underestimated because of unaccounted fetal demise, but it occurs in about 1 in 4,000–5,000 live births. Fetuses with large omphaloceles may benefit from cesarean sections to avoid injury to the herniated sac. Diagnosis is initiated by detection of increased levels of maternal serum alpha-fetoprotein and is confirmed by ultrasound. Shortly after delivery, there is a gradual surgical reduction of the visceral contents back into the abdominal cavity with a Silastic silo to cover the external gut in the interim. Complete reduction is not performed all at once in order to avoid excess intra-abdominal pressure and respiratory distress. Parenteral nutrition is used until the infant's gastrointestinal tract becomes functional.

Partial molar pregnancy. See Molar pregnancy.

Parvovirus—fifth disease. A DNA virus that can cause erythema infectiosum in children or hydrops fetalis in utero. There is only a 1% estimated chance of fetal infection in infected mothers, and there is no evidence of teratogenesis. Infected pregnant women may present with a rash that should prompt immediate attention. If she is found to have a positive blood test for a recent parvovirus infection, the pregnancy can be monitored more carefully with ultrasound and fetal testing. Many women already have had exposure to the parvovirus and have established immunity and are not at risk for fetal transmission.

Placental abruption (abruptio placentae). A separation of a normally implanted placenta, creating a hematoma (tumor of blood) that causes further separation. Ultimately, there is destruction of placental tissue in the involved area, thus decreasing the amount of tissue involved in respiratory gas exchange. Causes of abruption include trauma, maternal hypertension, cigarette smoking, high parity (number of previous pregnancies), and cocaine abuse. Symptoms include abdominal pain, uterine contractions and tenderness, and vaginal bleeding that is not proportional to the severity of the condition. Diagnosis is made by ultrasound. The pregnant woman should be hospitalized and her vital signs taken often, and an external fetal monitor should be placed. Complications include shock, damage to distant organs, and loss of the fetus.

Pneumothorax. A situation in which there is an accumulation of air in the pleural space. It may result from leakage of air from the lungs or airway, or more commonly from external trauma. Depending on the size, pneumothorax causes problems such as respiratory distress, which may present as cyanosis with physical exam signs of unilateral absent breath sounds, tracheal deviation, distended neck veins, and tympany to percussion of the involved side. Mechanical ventilation, asthma, cystic fibrosis, and disorders such as Marfan's syndrome predispose to this condition. Diagnosis is confirmed by X-ray, and treatment may require a chest tube (if the air collection is large) or needle aspiration, or no treatment may be needed. Infants born with respiratory distress as a result of prematurity and who need mechanical ventilation are at risk for pneumothorax as well as bronchopulmonary dysplasia from the high concentrations of external oxygen.

Posterior urethral valve obstruction. Though uncommon, it is the most common cause of bladder outlet obstruction in male infants. This condition causes dilation of the urethra and kidneys, and hypertrophy of the bladder walls. If the condition is severe in utero, oligohydramnios (too little amniotic fluid) is present and causes pulmonary hypoplasia. If less severe, it may present in the male infant as a urinary tract infection, weak urinary stream, and failure to thrive. Diagnosis is through ultrasound, and treatment includes decompression and valve ablation. Prognosis is good, but it depends upon whether the obstruction of the valve was severe in utero and the subsequent degree of urinary insufficiency.

Preterm labor and delivery. Defined as occurring after 20 weeks' and before 37 weeks' gestation with a changing cervix, preterm labor and delivery are associated with increased perinatal morbidity and mortality. Half of preterm labor and delivery cases are unexplained; the other half are associated with previous preterm labor and delivery, first trimester bleeding, urinary tract infections, multiple gestations, uterine anomalies, polyhydramnios, incompetent cervix, and medical reasons for induction, such as preeclampsia and uncontrolled third trimester bleeding with placenta previa or abruptio placenta. Low socioeconomic background of the mother seems to be an associated risk factor. Prevention includes identification of high-risk patients and early recognition of preterm contractions so that preterm labor can be stopped. Depending on the etiology, treatment of preterm labor includes placement in the left lateral decubitus position, close monitoring of both the mother and fetus through ultrasound, intravenous hydration, cervical cultures, blood work, urinalysis and tocolytic therapy to stop contractions if appropriate. Tocolytics include ritodrine, terbutaline, magnesium sulfate, prostaglandin synthesis inhibitors, and calcium channel blockers. Tocolysis usually delays delivery for more than seventy-two hours, enough time to administer glucocorticoid or thyroid-releasing hormone that will enhance pulmonary maturity of the fetus and decrease the incidence of neonatal respiratory distress syndrome. Preterm delivery needs careful assessment because the fetus often demonstrates malpresentation and is at greater risk for cord prolapse or compression. Because the head of a very preterm infant is proportionally much bigger than its body, breech delivery imposes the risk of head entrapment. Depending on the gestational age at birth, the infant is at increased risk of becoming septic, feeding problems, necrotizing enterocolitis, neonatal hypoglycemia, retinopathy, respiratory distress syndrome, intraventricular hemorrhage, seizures, sepsis, cerebral palsy, and mental retardation or learning disabilities.

Renal agenesis. Failure of development of one or both kidneys. Bilateral renal agenesis causes oligohydramnios (lack of amniotic fluid, which consists mostly of fetal urine). With lack of fluid, there is fetal compression by the uterus, which causes flat facies, clubfoot, and pulmonary hypoplasia (because lung development is dependent on amniotic fluid). This congregation of features is called Potter's syndrome, and these infants usually die of pulmonary insufficiency in the first week of life. Unilateral renal agenesis is often associated with reproductive tract abnormalities—for example, uterine anomalies such as uterus didelphys—due to the close interaction of these two systems during early fetal development. The existing kidney does a very good job of compensating with no or minimal decrease in renal function, so there is a normal life expectancy if the anomaly is not associated with other syndromes, such as VATER or Turner's.

Salpingitis isthmica nodosa. Also called tubal diverticulum, this condition is caused by the direct invasion of the muscular layer of the fallopian tube into the epithelial layer. This creates a higher chance for tubal (ectopic) pregnancy through disruption of transport of the fertilized ovum, rather than through mechanical obstruction.

Severe toxemia of pregnancy/preeclampsia/pregnancy-induced hypertension. A condition that usually occurs in the third trimester, but as late as 6 weeks postpartum, characterized by pathologic edema (fluid in the tissues of the hands and face rather than legs and feet), hypertension, and proteinuria. It most often affects younger patients in their first pregnancy and demonstrates a spectrum of severity judged by parameters of the hypertension and proteinuria. There are many proposed etiologies but none that is universally accepted. In addition to the above signs, there may be visual disturbances, hyperreflexia, and low platelet count. Management includes hospitalization, bed rest in the left lateral position to increase uterine blood flow, salt restriction, induction of labor if more than 36 weeks' gestation, antihypertensive medications (hydralazine) if the blood pressure is above 160/100, and anticonvulsant therapy (magnesium sulfate) administration during labor and delivery to prevent seizures. Caution must be exercised not to lower the blood pressure too quickly, in order to avoid decreased uteroplacental blood flow. There are no long-term maternal sequelae as long as there has been no cerebrovascular accident, a risk with any severe hypertensive episode. Infant sequelae are greater, especially if it is born preterm, because there are associated intrauterine growth retardation, fetal distress, and possible long-term central nervous system effects.

Short rib polydactyly syndrome. An autosomally recessive syndrome (requiring inheritance of two genes in order to manifest the disease) that comes in several forms, all of which demonstrate an infant having short ribs and polydactyly (extra digits on the hands or feet). This syndrome is typically incompatible with life because many viseral (internal organ) anomalies accompany the syndrome. Diagnosis is by ultrasound, which often reveals a hydropic infant.

Shoulder dystocia. Dystocia (difficult childbirth) refers to dysfunctional labor or labor that does not progress normally. It may be caused by disproportionate size of the fetus to the pelvis, as is the case in shoulder dystocia, in which the fetus's head comes out during delivery but progress of the delivery unexpectedly stops. Several maneuvers (e.g., McRoberts) must quickly be initiated to allow the anterior shoulder to pass from under the pubic symphysis, which is what is keeping the infant from being fully delivered. Another maneuver is added if the preceding one does not work, beginning with downward pressure on the suprapubic region, followed by flexion of the mother's thighs against the abdomen, episiotomy, pressure on the infant's scapula to turn the shoulder, insertion of the physician's hand into the vagina to pull the posterior arm across the chest, and last fracture of one or both of the infant's clavicles. There is definite potential for brachial plexus damage in the infant during these maneuvers, but the general health of the baby is in grave danger if they are not performed.

Spina bifida. This subgroup of neural tube defects has a wide range of severity. It is caused by failure of the neural tube to close during development, leaving an exposed area of tissue. The most severe is myelomeningocele, a mass of tissue that contains herniated spinal cord and its covering (meninges). Less severe is meningocele, which is a herniated mass containing only meninges. The least severe, and often asymptomatic, is spina bifida occulta, a vertebral defect without an associated herniation.

Staphylococcal (staph) infection. The *Staphylococcus* organism is part of the normal human flora in the nares (nostrils) of many asymptomatic people, and may be transmitted through nasal discharge, contaminated hands, and general contact. Newborns are very susceptible to this organism. It can affect almost every system, including the skin (as scalded skin syndrome or impetigo), the lungs (as pneumonia), the muscles (as abscesses), the bones and joints (as osteomyelitis and arthritis), the central nervous system (as meningitis and abscesses) the heart (as endocarditis, abscesses, and pericarditis), the kidneys (as abscesses), the intestinal tract (as food poisoning) and the entire body (as sepsis). Treatment includes antibiotics as well as incision and drainage of loculated collections of infected fluid. Staph toxin is the cause of toxic shock syndrome, which most often occurs in women using tampons and is characterized by abrupt onset, high fever, headache, vomiting, diarrhea, muscle aches, hypotension, rash, and shock. Mortality is about 3%.

Subchorionic hemorrhage. Hemorrhage that occurs between the chorion (outermost fetal membrane) and the decidual layer of the endometrium. It carries with it an increased risk of spontaneous abortion, intrapartum fetal demise, stillbirth, abruptio placenta, and preterm labor, especially with larger bleeds. The etiology of this type of hemorrhage is unknown.

GLOSSARY

Sudden infant death syndrome (SIDS). The unexpected death of an infant less than one year of age that cannot be explained. In the United States, it is the most common cause of death in the first year of life, with an incidence of approximately 1 to 2 per 1,000 live births. Recently it has been demonstrated that SIDS occurs more commonly in babies who sleep on their abdomens. Placing a baby on his or her back while sleeping may reduce the risk of SIDS. The pathology demonstrates hypoxia (lack of oxygen), and there are many proposed mechanisms, including aberrations in respiratory control and cardiac arrhythmias. No one theory is widely accepted.

Tay-Sachs disease. An autosomal recessive disease (requiring inheritance from both parents) in which there is a deficiency of an enzyme that leads to the destruction of neurons. There is an approximately 3% carrier frequency in Ashkenazi Jews, causing an incidence of about 1 in 3,600 of births. The disease, fatal in early childhood, is characterized by neurological degeneration (including severe mental retardation) and physical deterioration (including blindness that begins at about six months of age).

True knot. This is caused by entanglement of the umbilical cord, which occurs in less than 1% of all deliveries. In an otherwise normal umbilical cord, it is not thought to be the direct cause of fetal death. Therefore, further investigation should be employed in the event of fetal loss.

Twin-to-twin transfusion syndrome. A phenomenon that occurs as the result of an arterial-venous connection in the placenta, typically of monochorionic pregnancies, which leads to donation of blood from one twin that empties into the other twin. Due to this chronic shunting of blood, the donor twin demonstrates growth retardation, microcardia, hypovolemia, hypotension, and anemia, whereas the recipient twin may develop edema (fluid collection in tissues), cardiomegaly, hypervolemia, hypertension, and congestive heart failure. A key on ultrasound is oligohydramnios (too little amniotic fluid) in the donor twin's amniotic cavity and polyhydramnios (excess amniotic fluid) in that of the recipient. This condition carries significant morbidity and mortality, especially of the recipient twin. Treatment includes conservative management for mild twin-to-twin transfusion syndrome, and invasive therapies including serial or repetitive amniocentesis, laser photocoagulation and umbilical cord ligation for the more severe cases.

Uterine anomalies. Anatomical disturbances, either congenital or acquired, that are associated with pregnancy loss as well as with cervical incompetence. Uterine fibroids are acquired abnormalities that tend to occur in women in their late thirties and (more often) in black women. Surgical removal will increase the likelihood of carrying a pregnancy to term. Congenital anomalies usually occur as a consequence of malfusion during development and result in varying degrees of septation. The etiology is unknown, but it is believed to be from teratogens (e.g., DES exposure) in utero and/or genetic inheritance. Evaluation of these anomalies requires laparoscopy and hysteroscopy.

Vanishing twin syndrome. Death of one twin who was identified earlier in the pregnancy by ultrasound but is not found later in the pregnancy. There is an increased incidence of cerebral palsy in the surviving twin.

225

Vasa previa. Velamentous insertion of the umbilical cord where the unprotected vessels pass over the cervical os (opening), creating a greater risk of fetal vessel rupture. Once it is diagnosed, prompt abdominal delivery should be performed.

VATER syndrome. An acronym that describes the association of vertebral defects, anal atresia, tracheoesophageal fistula, and radial limb dysplasia. The etiology of this syndrome is unknown, and it falls under the category of sporadic syndrome complexes. Polyhydramnios secondary to tracheoesophageal fistula should cause intrapartum suspicion of this syndrome. After birth, coughing, choking, and cyanosis occur due to the fistula, so surgical repair is necessary. Congenital heart disease, usually ventricular septal defects, often accompanies this syndrome, as does unilateral renal agenesis.

Velamentous insertion of cord. Condition in which vessels of the umbilical cord insert between the amnion and chorion layers instead of in their normal insertion. This state incurs a greater risk of rupture of fetal vessels, which should prompt expedient abdominal delivery. The occurrence of velamentous insertion is higher in multiple pregnancies.

Volvulus. This occurs when the small intestine is not fixed in the abdomen, leading to twisting of the bowel that causes disruption of the blood supply, ischemia, and infarction. Abdominal pain, vomiting, diarrhea, and bloody stools are symptoms of this condition, and bowel perforation with peritonitis is a grave complication. A midgut volvulus is a surgical emergency.

NOTES

INTRODUCTION

1. M. Gordon, "A Moral Choice," *Atlantic Monthly* 265, no. 4: 78. Also in Walburga von Raffler-Engel, *The Perception of the Unborn across the Cultures of the World* (Toronto: Hogrefe and Huber, 1994), 105.

POETRY: COMFORTING THROUGH TIME

1. Czeslaw Milosz, *The Witness of Poetry* (Cambridge, MA: Harvard University Press, 1983), 25.

2. G. S. Rousseau, "Medicine and the Muses: An Approach to Literature and Medicine" in Marie Roberts and Roy Porter (eds.), *Literature and Medicine during the Eighteenth Century* (London: Routledge, 1993).

3. John Fox, *Poetic Medicine: The Healing Art of Poem-Making* (New York: Jeremy P. Tarcher/Penguin Putnam, 1997), 5.

4. Irwin Edman, *The World, the Arts and the Artist* (New York: W. W. Norton, 1928), 30.

5. Mary Jane Moffat, *In the Midst of Winter* (New York: Vintage Books, 1992), xxiv.

6. Rita Dove, in Fox, *Poetic Medicine*, 4.

7. Lisel Mueller, in Stephen Kuusisto, Deborah Tall, and David Weiss, eds., *The Poet's Notebook* (New York: W. W. Norton, 1995), 215.

8. Moffat, *In the Midst of Winter*, xxiv.

9. "Poetry is rhythmical. Rhythm secures the heightening of physiological consciousness so as to shut out sensory perception of the environment. In the rhythm of dance, music or song we become self conscious instead of conscious. The rhythm of a heartbeat and breathing and physiological periodicity negates the physical rhythm of the environment." Christopher Caudwell, in Melvin Rader, *A Modern Book of Aesthetics* (New York: Holt, Rinehart and Winston, 1965), 154.

10. D. H. Lawrence, in Stewart L. Udall, *The Quiet Crisis* (New York: Holt, Rinehart, and Winston, 1963), 1.

11. Randall White, *Dark Caves, Bright Visions: Life in Ice Age Europe* (New York: American Museum of Natural History/W. W. Norton,), 19.

12. Ibid., 14.

13. Ibid., 19.

14. Ibid.

15. Rader, *A Modern Book of Aesthetics*, 155.

16. Edman, *The World, the Arts and the Artist*, 30.

17. Ibid.

18. Emanuel Feldman, *Biblical and Post-Biblical Defilement and Mourning: Law as Theology* (New York: Yeshiva University Press/KTAV Publishing House, 1977), 3.

19. Dr. Palmer Findley, *The Story of Childbirth* (New York: Doubleday, 1934), 2.

20. Observed at American Museum of Natural History, New York.

21. Ralph S. Solecki, *Shanidar: The First Flower People* (New York: Alfred A. Knopf, 1971), 247.

22. Edward Burnett Tylor, in White, *Dark Caves, Bright Visions*, 14.

23. Marija Gimbutas, *The Language of the Goddess* (San Francisco: HarperCollins, 1991), 316.

24. Ibid.

25. Ibid., xvii.

26. Ibid., 213.

27. Andre Leroi-Gourhan, in White, *Dark Caves, Bright Visions*, 157.

28. Douglas J. Davies, *Death, Ritual and Belief: The Rhetoric of Funerary Rites* (London: Cassell, 1997), 133.

29. Bernardo T. Arriaza, *Beyond Death: The Chinchorro Mummies of Ancient Chile* (Washington, DC: Smithsonian Institution Press, 1995), 139.

30. Davies, *Death, Ritual and Belief*, 132–133.

31. Richard Deurer, *Egypt and Art*, http://m2.aol.com/egyptart/hathor.html (WWW page, January 1997).

32. *The Papyrus of Ani* (240 B.C.), trans. E. A. Wallis Budge (New York: Dover Publications, 1967), 188.

33. Findley, *The Story of Childbirth*, 155.

34. Ibid., 274.

35. Darrel W. Amundsen, *Medicine, Society and Faith in the Ancient and Medieval Worlds* (Baltimore: Johns Hopkins University Press, 1996), 52.

36. Ibid.

37. John M. Rist, *Human Value: A Study in Ancient Philosophical Ethics*, cited in Amundsen, *Medicine, Society, and Faith*, 52.

38. Heliodorus, *An Ethiopian Romance*, trans. Moses Hadas (Ann Arbor: University of Michigan Press, 1957), 61.

39. Findley, *The Story of Childbirth*, 274.

40. Ibid., 165.

41. Christopher Daniell, *Death and Burial in Medieval England, 1066–1550* (London: Routledge, 1997), 124–125.

42. Ibid., 125–126.

43. Ibid., 127.

44. Rabbi Debra Orenstein, *Life Cycles: Jewish Women on Life Passages and Personal Milestones*, vol. 1 (Woodstock, VT: Jewish Lights, 1994), 37.

45. Colin Murray Parkes, Pittu Laungani, and Bill Young, *Death and Bereavement across Cultures* (London: Routledge, 1997), 194.

46. Ibid.

CHERISHED PURPOSES: SELECTIONS FROM A DOCTOR'S POEMS

1. Elie Wiesel, The Nobel Lecture: Hope, Despair and Memory in the *Nobel Peace Prize 1986* (New York: Summit Books, 1986), 21.

2. Thomas A. Dooley, M.D., *The Night They Burned the Mountain* (New York: Signet Books, 1960), 32.

3. Lisel Mueller in Stephen Kuusisto, Deborah Tall, and David Weiss, *The Poet's Notebook: Excerpts from the Notebooks of Contemporary American Poets* (New York: W.W. Norton and Company, 1995), 215

4. Douglas J. Davies, *Death, Ritual and Belief: The Rhetoric of Funerary Rites* (Washington, D.C.: Cassell, 1997), 1.

5. Irwin Edman *The World, the Arts and the Artist* (New York: W.W. Norton & Company, Inc. 1928), 30

6. Edman, *The World, the Arts and the Artist*, 51.

7. Mueller, *The Poet's Notebook*, 215.

PARENTS' STORIES OF LOSS

1. Francis Ridley Havergal, in Michele Durkson Clise, *Memento: Solace for Grieving* (Boston: Little, Brown, 1995), 5.

2. Michael R. Berman, M.D., *Hygeia: An Online Journal for Pregnancy and Neonatal Loss* (1998). Available from http://www.hygeia.org.

3. SHARE (Source of Help in Airing and Resolving Experiences), a paradigm for perinatal support groups, was funded in 1977.

4. Lucian Pye, *Communications and Political Development* (Princeton, NJ: Princeton University Press, 1963), 4.

5. Mark Poster, *The Mode of Information* (Chicago: University of Chicago Press, 1990), 116.

6. Michael R. Berman, M.D., *Hygeia: An Online Journal for Pregnancy and Neonatal Loss* (1998). Available from http://www.hygeia.org.

REASONS FOR THE MOST COMMON PERINATAL LOSSES

1. A. H. Handyside, J. K. Pattinson, R. J. Penketh, J. D. Delhanty, R. M. Winston, and E. G. Tuddenham, Biopsy of human preimplantation embryos and sexing by DNA amplification. *Lancet* (1989); 347–349:8634; A. Dokras, I. L. Sargent, C. Ross, R. L. Gardner, and D. H. Barlow, Trophectoderm biopsy in human blastocysts. *Hum Reprod* (1990); 5(7):821–825.

2. L. F. Goncalves, R. Romero, M. Silva, F. Ghezzi, A. Soto, H. Munoz, and A. Ghidini, Reverse flow in the ductus venosus: An ominous sign, *American Journal of Obstetrics and Gynecology* (1995); 172(1): 266 (abstr. 33).

3. M. Toppozada, N. Sallam, A. Gaffar, et al. Role of repeated stretching in the mechanism of timely rupture of the membranes. *American Journal of Obstetrics and Gynecology* (1970); 108:243.

4. N. Kanayama, and T.Y.K. Terao. Collagen types in normal prematurely ruptured amniotic membranes. *American Journal of Obstetrics and Gynecology* (1985); 153:899; F. Vadillo-Ortega, G. Gonzalez-Avilla, S. Karclimen, et al. Collagen metabolism in premature rupture of amniotic membranes. *Obstetrics and Gynecology* (1990); 75:84.

5. R. Naeye. Factors that predispose to premature rupture of membranes. *Obstetrics and Gynecology* (1982); 60:93; J. H. Harger, A. Hsing, R. Tuomola, et al. Risk factors for preterm premature rupture of fetal membranes: A multicenter case-control study. *American Journal of Obstetrics and Gynecology* (1990); 163:130; C. Hadley, D. Main, and S. Gabbe. Risk factors for preterm premature rupture of fetal membranes. *American Journal of Perinatology* (1990); 7:374.

6. P. B. Mead. Management of the patient with premature rupture of the membranes. *Clinics in Perinatology* (1980); 7:243–255; T. J. Garite, R. K. Freeman, E. M. Linzey, P. S. Braly, and W. L. Dorchester. Prospective randomized study of corticosteroids in the management of premature rupture of the membranes and the premature gestation. *American Journal of Obstetrics and Gynecology* (1981); 141: 508–515.

7. T. Garite and R. K. Freeman. Chorioamnionitis in the preterm gestation. *Obstetrics and Gynecology* (1982); 54:539; R. S. Bibbs, J. D. Blanco, P. J. St. Clair, et al. Quantitative bacteriology of amniotic fluid from patients with clinical intra-amniotic infection at term. *Journal of Infectious Diseases* (1982); 145:1.

8. C. C. Gunn, D. R. Mishell, and D. G. Morton. Premature rupture of the fetal membranes. *American Journal of Obstetrics and Gynecology* (1970); 106:469.

9. S. E. Rutherford, J. P. Phelan, C. V. Smith, and N. Jacobs. The four quadrant assessment of amniotic fluid volume: An adjunct to antepartum fetal heart rate testing. *Obstetrics and Gynecology* (1987); 70:353; S. G. Gabbe, B. B. Ettinger, R. K. Freeman, et al. Umbilical cord compression associated with amniotomy: Laboratory observations. *American Journal of Obstetrics and Gynecology* (1976); 126:353.

10. L. Moberg and T. Garite. Antepartum fetal heart rate testing in preterm PROM. Presented at Seventh Annual Meeting of the Society of Perinatal Obstetricians, Lake Buena, FL, 1987.

11. A. M. Vintzileos, W. A. Campbell, D. J. Nochimson, and P. J. Weinbaum. Degree of oligohydramnios and pregnancy outcome in patients with premature rupture of the membranes. *Obstetrics and Gynecology* (1985); 66:162.

12. K. Itoh and H. Itoh. A study of cartilage development in pulmonary hypoplasia. *Pediatric Pathology* (1988); 8:65.

13. A. Rotschild, E. W. Ling, M. L. Puterman, et al. Neonatal outcome after prolonged preterm rupture of the membranes. *American Journal of Obstetrics and Gynecology* (1990); 162:46; C. Nimrod, F. Varela-Gittings, G. Machin, et al. The effect of very prolonged membrane rupture on fetal development. *American Journal of Obstetrics and Gynecology* (1984); 148:540.

14. P. Vergani, A. Ghidini, A. Locatelli, et al. Risk factors for pulmonary hypoplasia in second trimester PROM. *American Journal of Obstetrics and Gynecology* (1994); 170:1359.

15. C. Nimrod, D. Davies, S. Iwanleki, et al. Ultrasound prediction of pulmo-

nary hypoplasia. *Obstetrics and Gynecology* (1986); 68:495; A. M. Vintzileos, W. A. Campbell, J. F. Rodis, et al. Comparison of six different ultrasonographic methods for predicting lethal fetal pulmonary hypoplasia. *American Journal of Obstetrics and Gynecology* (1989); 161:606.

16. M.J. Keirse, A. Ohlsson, P. E. Treffers, and H.H.H. Kanhai. Prelabour rupture of membranes preterm. In I. Chalmers, M. Enkin, and M. J. Keirse, eds., *Effective Care in Pregnancy and Childbirth*, 666–693. Oxford: Oxford University Press, 1989.

17. B. M. Mercer and K. L. Arheart. Antimicrobial therapy in the expectant management of preterm premature rupture of membranes. *Lancet* (1995); 346:1271.

18. P. A. Crowley, I. Chalmers, and M. J. Keirse. The effects of corticosteroid administration before preterm delivery: An overview of evidence from controlled trials. *British Journal of Obstetrics and Gynaecology* (1990); 97:11.

19. P. A. Crowley. Corticosteroids prior to preterm delivery. In *Oxford Database of Perinatal Trials*. Oxford: Oxford University Press, 1992.

20. C. R. Bauer, C. Morrison, et al. A decreased incidence of necrotizing enterocolitis after prenatal glucocorticoid therapy. *Pediatrics* (1984); 73:682.

21. P. B. Mead. Management of the patient with premature rupture of the membranes. *Clinics in Perinatology* (1980); 7:243–255.

22. K. K. Christensen, I. Ingemarsson, T. Leideman, H. Solum, and N. Svenningsen. Effect of ritodrine on labor after premature rupture of the membranes. *Obstetrics and Gynecology* (1980); 55:155; T. J. Garite, K. A. Keegan, R. K. Freeman, and M. P. Nageotte. A randomized trial of ritodrine tocolysis versus expectant management in patients with premature rupture of membranes at 25 to 30 weeks of gestation. *American Journal of Obstetrics and Gynecology* (1987); 157:388; C. P. Weiner, K. Renk, and M. Klugman. The therapeutic efficacy and cost effectiveness of aggressive tocolysis for premature labor associated with premature rupture of the membranes. *American Journal of Obstetrics and Gynecology* (1988); 159:216.

23. D. L. Levy and S. L. Warsof. Oral ritodrine and preterm premature rupture of membranes. *Obstetrics and Gynecology* (1985); 66:621; P.D.M. Dunlop, P. A. Crowley, R. F. Lamont, and D. F. Hawkins. Preterm ruptured membranes, no contractions. *Journal of Obstetrics and Gynaecology* (1986); 7:92–96.

24. M. E. Hannah, C. M. Ohisson, D. Farine, S. A. Hewson, et al. Induction of labor compared with expectant management for prelabor rupture of the membranes at term. *New England Journal of Medicine* (1996); 334:1005.

25. T. Garite and R. K. Freeman. Chorioamnionitis in the preterm gestation. *Obstetrics and Gynecology* (1982); 54:539.

26. E. C. Hughes, ed. *Obstetric-Gynecologic Terminology*. Philadelphia: F. A. Davis, 1972.

27. E. W. Page and R. Christianson. The impact of mean arterial blood pressure in the middle trimester upon outcome of pregnancy. *American Journal of Obstetrics and Gynecology* (1976); 125:740.

28. O. Talledo, L. C. Chesley, and F. P. Zuspan. Renin-angiotensin system in normal and toxemic pregnancies. III. Differential sensitivity to angiotensin II and norepinephrine in toxemia of pregnancy. *American Journal of Obstetrics and Gynecology* (1968); 100:218.

29. N. F. Gant, G. L. Daley, S. Chand, et al. A study of angiotensin II pressor

response throughout primigravid pregnancy. *Journal of Clinical Investigation* (1973); 52:2682.

30. F. G. Cunningham and M. D. Lindeheimer. Hypertension in pregnancy. *New England Journal of Medicine* (1992); 326:927.

31. C. Dadak, A. Kefalides, H. Sinzinger, and G. Weber. Reduced umbilical artery prostacyclin formation in complicated pregnancies. *American Journal of Obstetrics and Gynecology* (1982); 144:792.

32. S. Moncada, R.M.I. Palmer, and E. A. Higgs. Nitric oxide: Physiology, pathophysiology, and pharmacology. *Pharmacology Review* (1991); 43:109.

33. L. C. Chesley. *Hypertensive Disorders in Pregnancy.* New York: Appleton-Century-Crofts, 1978.

34. C.W.G. Redman, L. J. Beilin, and J. Bonnar. Plasma urate measurement in predicting fetal death in hypertensive pregnancies. *Lancet* (1976); 1:1370.

35. J. A. Pritchard, F. G. Cunningham, and R. A. Mason. Coagulation changes in eclampsia: Their frequency and pathogenesis. *American Journal of Obstetrics and Gynecology* (1976); 124:855.

36. L. Weinstein. Syndrome of hemolysis, elevated liver enzymes, and low platelet count: A severe consequence of hypertension in pregnancy. *American Journal of Obstetrics and Gynecology* (1982); 142:159.

37. B. M. Sibai, M. M. Taslimi, A. El-Nazar, et al. Maternal-perinatal outcome associated with the syndrome of hemolysis, elevated liver enzymes, and low platelets in severe preeclampsia-eclampsia. *American Journal of Obstetrics and Gynecology* (1986); 155:501.

38. T. Y. Khong, F. De Wolf, W. B. Robertson, and I. Brosens. Inadequate maternal response to placentation in pregnancies complicated by pre-eclampsia and by small-gestational age infants. *British Journal of Obstetrics and Gynaecology* (1986); 93:1049.

39. J. L. Kitzmiller and K. Benirschke. Immunofluorescent study of placental bed vessels in pre-eclampsia. *American Journal of Obstetrics and Gynecology* (1973); 115:248.

40. J. A. Pritchard and S. R. Stone. Clinical and laboratory observations on eclampsia. *American Journal of Obstetrics and Gynecology* (1967); 99:754.

41. T. F. Imperiale and A. S. Petrulis. A meta-analysis of low-dose aspirin for the prevention of pregnancy-induced hypertensive disease. *Journal of the American Medical Association* (1991); 266:261.

42. P. F. Plouin, G. Chatellier, G. Breart, et al. Frequency and perinatal consequences of hypertensive disease of pregnancy. *Advances in Nephrology* (1986); 57: 69.

43. R. L. Naeye and E. A. Friedman. Causes of perinatal death associated with gestational hypertension and proteinuria. *American Journal of Obstetrics and Gynecology* (1979); 133:8.

44. L. Tervila, G. Goecke, and S. Timonen. Estimation of gestosis of pregnancy (ERH-gestosis). *Acta Obstetrica et Gynecologica Scandinavica* (1973); 52:235.

45. N. J. Sebire, S. Thornton, K. Hughes, R. J. Snijders, and K. H. Nicolaides. The prevalence and consequences of missed abortion in twin pregnancies at 10 to 14 weeks of gestation. *British Journal of Obstetrics and Gynaecology* (1997); 104: 847–48.

46. P. Schreiner-Engel, V. N. Walther, J. Mindes, L. Lynch, and R. L. Berkow-

itz. First-trimester multifetal pregnancy reduction: Acute and persistent psychologic reactions. *American Journal of Obstetrics and Gynecology* (1995); 172:541–47.

47. J. W. Ballantyne. The problem of the postmature infant. *Journal of Obstetrics and Gynaecology of the British Empire* (1902); 2(36):521–544.

48. S. H. Clifford. Postmaturity—with placenta dysfunction. *Journal of Pediatrics* (1954); 44:1.

49. R. Hasseljo and A. C. Auberg. Prolonged pregnancy. *Acta Obstetrics and Gynaecology of Scandinavia Supplementary* (1962); 61:23–29.

50. J. T. Lanman. Delays during reproduction and their effects on the embryo and fetus. *New England Journal of Medicine* (1968); 278:1092–1099.

51. P. Bergsjo. Postterm pregnancy: Induction or surveillance. In *Progress in Obstetrics and Gynaecology*, vol. 5, J. W. Studd, ed., 121–133. Edinburgh and London: Churchill Livingstone, 1985.

52. P. Crowley. Post term pregnancy: Induction or surveillance. In I. Chalmers, M. Enkin, and M. J. Keirse, eds., *Effective Care in Pregnancy and Childbirth*, 776–791 Oxford: Oxford University Press, 1989.

53. Ibid.

54. V. A. Barss, F. D. Frigoletto, and F. Diamond. Stillbirth after nonstress testing. *Obstetrics and Gynecology* (1985); 65:541; M. E. Boyd, R. H. Usher, F. H. McLean, et al. Obstetric consequences of post-maturity. *American Journal of Obstetrics and Gynecology* (1988); 158:334.

55. World Health Organization. Recommended definitions, terminology and format for statistical tables related to the perinatal period and use of a new certificate for cause of perinatal deaths. *Acta Obstetrics and Gynecology Scandinavia* (1977); 56: 247–253.

56. International Federation of Gynecology and Obstetrics. FIGO news: List of gynecologic and obstetrical terms and definitions. *International Journal of Gynecology and Obstetrics* (1976); 14:570–576.

57. L. Bakketeig and P. Bergsjo. Postterm pregnancy: Magnitude of the problem. In I. Chalmers, M. Enkin and M. J. Keirse, eds., *Effective Care in Pregnancy and Childbirth*, 765–775. Oxford: Oxford University Press, 1989.

58. Crowley, Post term pregnancy.

59. N. Saunders and C. Paterson. Can we abandon Naegele's rule? *Lancet* (1991); 337:600–601.

60. R. Mittendorf, M. A. Williams, and C. S. Berkey. The length of uncomplicated human gestation. *Obstetrics and Gynecology* (1990); 75:929–932.

61. H. B. Mere. Ultrasound demonstration of an unusual fetal growth pattern in Indians. *British Journal of Obstetrics and Gynaecology* (1981); 88:260–263.

62. G. Von Doring. Über die Tragzeit post Ovulation: Geburtshilfe. *Frauenheilkd* (1962); 22:1191–1194.

63. J. Gardosi and M. Mongelli. Risk assessment adjusted for gestational age in maternal serum screening for Down's syndrome. *British Medical Journal* (1993); 306:1509–1511.

64. H. P. Robinson and J. E. Fleming, A critical evaluation of crown-rump length measurement. *British Journal Of Obstetrics and Gynaecology* (1975); 82:702–710.

65. S. Campbell and G. B. Newman. Growth of the fetal biparietal diameter

during normal pregnancy. *Journal of Obstetrics and Gynaecology of the British Commonwealth* (1971); 78:513–519.

66. M. H. Hall. Definitions used in relation to gestational age. *Paediatric Perinatal Epidemiology* (1990); 4:123–128.

67. P. H. Persson and B. M. Weldner. Reliability of ultrasound fetometry in estimating gestational age in the second trimester. *Acta Obstetrics et Gynaecology Scandinavia* (1986); 65:481–483.

68. M. Mongelli and B. Opatola. Duration and variability of normal pregnancy: Implication for clinical practice. *Journal of Reproductive Medicine* (1995); 40(9): 645–648.

69. M. Mongelli, M. Wilcox, and J. Gardosi. Estimating the date of confinement: Ultrasonographic biometry versus certain menstrual dates. *American Journal of Obstetrics and Gynecology* (1996); 174(1):278–281.

70. WHO. Recommended definitions, terminology and format for statistical tables.

71. R. T. Geirsson and R.M.C. Busby-Earle. Certain dates may not provide a reliable estimate of gestational age. *British Journal of Obstetrics and Gynaecology* (1991); 98:108–109.

72. U. Waldenstroem, O. Axelson, and S. Nilsson. A comparison of the ability of a sonographically measured biparietal diameter and the last menstrual period to predict the spontaneous onset of labor. *Obstetrics and Gynecology* (1990); 76:336–338.

73. Geirsson and Busby-Earle. Certain dates may not provide a reliable estimate of gestational age.

74. Mongelli, Wilcox, and Gardosi. Estimating the date of confinement.

75. M. E. Hannah. Postterm pregnancy: Should all women have labor induced? A review of literature. *Fetal Maternal Medicine Review* (1993); 5:3–17.

76. M. E. Hannah, W. J. Hannah, J. Hellman, et al. Induction of labor as compared with serial antenatal monitoring in postterm pregnancy: A randomized controlled trial. *New England Journal of Medicine* (1992); 326:1587–1592.

77. J. Shime et al. Prolonged pregnancy surveillance of the fetus and the neonate and the course of labor and delivery. *American Journal of Obstetrics and Gynecology* (1984); 148:547–552.

78. E. Sadovsky and H. Yaffe. Daily fetal movement recording and fetal prognosis. *Obstetrics and Gynecology* (1973); 41:845–850.

79. A. Grant et al. Routine fetal movement counting and risk of antepartum late death in normally formed singletons. *Lancet* (1989); 2:346–349.

80. Hannah, Postterm pregnancy.

81. N. A. Beischer, J. H. Evans, and L. Townsend. Studies in prolonged pregnancy: The incidence of prolonged pregnancy. *American Journal of Obstetrics and Gynecology* (1969); 103:476–482.

82. T. R. Moore and J. E. Cayle. Amniotic fluid index in normal human pregnancy. *American Journal of Obstetrics and Gynecology* (1990); 162:1168; A. D. Marks and M. Y. Divon. Longitudinal study of the amniotic fluid index in postdates pregnancy. *Obstetrics and Gynecology* (1992); 79:29–33.

83. K. J. Trimmer et al. Observations on the cause of oligohydramnios in prolonged pregnancy. *American Journal of Obstetrics and Gynecology* (1990); 163:1900–1903.

84. P. Crowley, C. O'Herlihy, and P. Boylan. The value of ultrasound measurement of amniotic volume in the management of prolonged pregnancies. *British Journal of Obstetrics and Gynaecology* (1984); 91:444–448.

85. S. E. Rutherford et al. The four quadrant assessment of amniotic fluid volume: An adjunct to antepartum fetal heart rate testing. *Obstetrics and Gynecology* (1997); 70:353.

86. J. N. Martin et al. Alternative approaches to the management of gravidas with prolonged postterm pregnancies. *Journal of the Mississippi State Medical Association* (1989); 30:105–111; A. L. Medearis. Postterm pregnancy: Active induction (PGE2gel) not associated with improved outcomes compared to expectant management: A preliminary report. In *Proceedings of 10th annual meeting of the Society of Perinatal Obstetricians 1990*. Houston, TX; A. M. Suikkari et al. Prolonged pregnancy: Induction or observation? *Acta Obstetrics et Gynecology Scandinavia* (1983); 116(suppl.):58.

87. J. N. Green and R. H. Paul. The value of amniocentesis in prolonged pregnancy. *Obstetrics, and Gynecology* (1978); 51:293–298.

88. Z. Katz et al. Nonaggressive management of postdate pregnancies. *European Journal of Obstetrics, Gynecology and Reproductive Biology* (1983); 15:71–79.

89. G. E. Knox et al. Management of prolonged pregnancy: Results of a prospective randomized trial. *American Journal of Obstetrics and Gynecology* (1979); 134:376–381.

90. L. D. Devoe and J. S. Scholl. Post date pregnancy: Assessment of fetal risk and obstetric management. *Journal of Reproductive Medicine* (1983); 28(9):676–80.

91. J. L. Small, J. P. Phelan, S. V. Smith et al. An active management approach to the postdate fetus with a reactive nonstress test in fetal heart rate decelerations. *Obstetrics and Gynecology* (1967); 70:636.

92. P. Mohide and M. J. Keirse. Biophysical assessment of fetal well-being: In I. Chalmers, M. Enkin, and M. J. Keirse, eds., *Effective Care in Pregnancy and Childbirth*, vol. 1, 477–492. Oxford: Oxford University Press, 1989.

93. R. L. Fischer et al. Doppler evaluation of umblical and uterine arcuate arteries in the postdates pregnancies. *Obstetrics and Gynecology* (1991); 78:363–368.

94. H. J. Stokes, R. V. Roberts, and J. P. Newham. Doppler flow velocity waveform analysis in postdates pregnancies. *Australian and New Zealand Journal of Obstetrics and Gynaecology* (1991); 81:27–30.

95. M. J. Keirse and A. C. A. van Oppen. Preparing the cervix for induction of labour. In I. Chalmers, M. Enkin, and M. J. Keirse, eds., *Effective Care in Pregnancy and Childbirth*, 988–1056. Oxford: Oxford University Press, 1989.

96. H. Vorherr. Placental insufficiency in relation to postterm pregnancy and fetal postmaturity: Evaluation of fetoplacental function: Management of the postterm gravida. *European Journal of Obstetrics, Gynecology and Reproductive Biology* (1974); 123:67–100.

97. D. C. Dyson. Fetal surveillance vs labor induction at 42 weeks in postterm gestation. *Journal of Reproductive Medicine* (1988); 33:262–270.

98. R. K. Freeman et al. Utilization of contraction stress testing for primary fetal surveillance. *American Journal of Obstetrics and Gynecology* (1981); 140:128–135.

99. L. D. Cardozo, J. Fysh, and J. M. Pearse. Prolonged pregnancy: The management debate. *British Medical Journal* (1986); 293:1059–1063; P. Bergsjo et al.

Comparison of induced versus non-induced labor in postterm pregnancy: A randomized prospective study. *Acta Obstetrics et Gynecology Scandinvia* (1989); 68:683–687.

100. R. Goeree, M. Hannah, S. Hewson et al. Cost effectiveness of induction of labour versus serial antenatal monitoring in the Canadian Multicenter Postterm Pregnancy trial. *Canadian Medical Association Journal* (1995); 152(9):1445–1450.

101. M. E. Hannah. Management of postterm pregnancy. *Journal of the Society of Obstetricians and Gynaecologists of Canada* (1994); 4:1581–1591.

102. Cardozo, Fysh, and Pearse. Prolonged pregnancy.

103. L. J. Roberts and K. R. Young. The management of prolonged pregnancy—An analysis of women's attitudes before and after term. *British Journal of Obstetrics and Gynaecology* (1991); 98:1102–1106.

REFLECTIONS

1. A personal eulogy delivered at a memorial service for stillborn babies buried in a mass burial site.

2. Octavio Paz in John Fox, *Poetic Medicine: The Healing Art of Poem Making* (New York: Jeremy P. Tarcher/Putnam, 1997), 48.

3. Tom Dooley, *The Night They Burned the Mountain* (Cutchogue, NY: Buccaneer Books, 1993), 19.

4. John Donne, *Devotions upon Emergent Occasions* (1624).

5. Elie Wiesel, "A Song for Hope," in Carol Rittner, *Elie Wiesel: Between Memory and Hope* (New York: New York University Press, 1990), 208.

SELECTED BIBLIOGRAPHY

American College of Obstetrics and Gynecology. *Substance Abuse*. Technical Bulletin no. 194 (July 1994).

Aristotle. *Poetics*. Translated by Gerald F. Else. Ann Arbor: University of Michigan Press, 1970.

Arnold, Joan Hagan, and Gemma, Penelope Buschman. *A Child Dies: A Portrait of Family Grief*, 2nd ed. Philadelphia: Charles Press, 1994.

Bell, Gil., and Lau, K. "Perinatal and Neonatal Issues of Substance Abuse." *Pediatric Clinics of North America* 42 (2) (1995):261–281.

Benson, Judi, and Falk, Agneta. *The Long Pale Corridor: Contemporary Poems of Bereavement*. Newcastle upon Tyne, UK: Bloodaxe Books, 1996.

Bluenfeld-Kosinski, Renate. *Not of Woman Born: Representations of Caesarean Birth in Medieval and Renaissance Culture*. Ithaca, NY: Cornell University Press, 1990.

Blum, Jeffrey. *Living with Spirit in a Material World*. New York: Ballantine Books, 1981.

Cacciatore, Joanne. *Dear Cheyenne: A Journey into Grief*. Peoria, Mothers in Sympathy and Support, 1996.

Faldet, Rachel, and Fitton, Karen. *Our Stories of Miscarriage: Healing with Words*. Minneapolis: Fairview Press, 1997.

Fertig, Mona. *A Labor of Love: An Anthology of Poetry on Pregnancy and Childbirth*. Winlaw, Polestar Press, 1989.

Hacker, N. F., and Moore, J. G. *Essentials of Obstetrics and Gynecology*, 2nd ed. Philadelphia: W. B. Saunders, 1992.

Hawkes, Jacquetta, and Woolley, Sir Leonard. *History of Mankind*, vol. 1, *Prehistory and the Beginnings of Civilization*. New York: Harper & Row, 1963.

Hickerson, Nancy Parrott. *Linguistic Anthropology*. Orlando, FL: Harcourt Brace Jovanovich College Publishers, 1980.

Kluge, Eike-Henner W. *The Practice of Death*. New Haven, CT: Yale University Press, 1975.

Kohn, Ingrid, and Moffitt, Perry-Lynn. *A Silent Sorrow: Pregnancy Loss.* New York: Delacorte Press, 1992.

Lafser, Christine O'Keeffe. *An Empty Cradle, A Full Heart: Reflections for Mothers and Fathers after Miscarriage, Stillbirth, or Infant Death.* Chicago: Loyola Press, 1998.

Lammert, Cathi, and Friedeck, Sue. *Angelic Presence: Short Stories of Solace and Hope after the Loss of a Baby.* Salt Lake City: Richard Paul Evans, 1997.

Little, B. B., and Van Beveren, T. T. "Placental Transfer of Selected Substances of Abuse." *Seminars in Perinatology* 20 (2) (1996):147–153.

Lothrop, Hannah. *Help, Comfort and Hope after Losing Your Baby in Pregnancy or the First Year.* Tucson, AZ: Fisher Books, 1997.

Mueller, Lisel. *Alive Together: New and Selected Poems.* Baton Rouge: Louisiana State University Press, 1986.

Murray, Thomas H. *The Worth of a Child.* Berkeley: University of California Press, 1996.

Otten, Charlotte. *The Virago Book of Birth Poetry.* London: Virago Press, 1993.

Rich, Laurie A. *When Pregnancy Isn't Perfect.* New York: Penguin Group, 1993.

Tiger, Lionel. *Optimism: The Biology of Hope.* New York: Simon and Schuster, 1979.

Wheeler, S. F. "Substance Abuse during Pregnancy." *Primary Care* 20 (1) (1993): 191–207.

INTERNET WEBSITES

A Heartbreaking Choice: http://www.erichad.com/ahc/

Arizona SIDS Alliance: http://azsids.org/

CDC Reproductive Health Information: http://www.cdc.gov/nccdphp/drh/art.htm

The Compassionate Friends: http://www.compassionatefriends.org/

The Genetic Alliance: http://www.geneticalliance.org/

Genetics and IVF Institute: http://www.givf.com/

Growth House, Inc.: http://www.growthhouse.org/

Hygeia.org; A Journal for parenthood lost; Michael R. Berman, M.D.: http://www.hygeia.org

The InterNational Council on Infertility Information Dissemination: http://www.inciid.org

IVF.COM: http://www.ivf.com/

March of Dimes: http://www.modimes.org/

National Organization for Rare Diseases: http://www.rarediseases.org/

Resolve: http://www.resolve.org/

SANDS Australia: http://www.sands.org.au/

SHARE: http://www.nationalshareoffice.com/

Support Organization for Trisomy 18, 13 and other Related Disorders: http://www.trisomy.org/

WiSSP; Wisconsin Stillbirth Service Program: http://www.wisc.edu/wissp/

INDEX

CONTRIBUTORS

Karen Aresco, parent and caregiver

Kristen Aversa, MD, medical student, Yale University School of Medicine

Brenda Whiting Beard, R.N., BSN, Nurse, Labor and Delivery Suite, Yale-New Haven Hospital, and Codirector, Maternity Bereavement Services, Yale-New Haven Hospital

Louise Cerrone Bell, parent

Julia Bishop-Hahlo, R.N., Newborn Special Care Unit, Yale-New Haven Hospital

Frank H. Boehm, MD, Professor and Director of Maternal/Fetal Medicine, Vanderbilt University Medical Center

Adina Chelouche, MD, Instructor, Department of Obstetrics and Gynecology, Yale University School of Medicine

Leslie Ciarlegio, MS, certified genetic counselor, Perinatal Unit, Yale-New Haven Hospital

Joshua A. Copel, MD, Professor of Obstetrics and Gynecology, Yale University School of Medicine, and Director of Obstetrics, Yale-New Haven Hospital

Anuja Dokras, MD, PhD, Fellow in Reproductive Endocrinology, Department of Obstetrics and Gynecology, Yale University School of Medicine

Steven J. Fleischman, MD, Resident in Obstetrics and Gynecology, Yale-New Haven Hospital

Jennifer Goins-Caufman, parent

Laurel Jonason, R.N., BSN, Nurse, Newborn Special Care Unit, and Co-director, Perinatal Bereavement Services, Yale-New Haven Hospital

David Jones, MD, Associate Professor, Department of Obstetrics and Gynecology, Section of Maternal and Fetal Medicine, Yale University School of Medicine

Ande L. Karimu, MD, PhD, Resident, Department of Obstetrics and Gynecology, Yale-New Haven Hospital

Harvey J. Kliman, MD, PhD, Placental Pathologist, Department of Obstetrics and Gynecology, Yale University School of Medicine

David Lima, MD, Instructor, Department of Obstetrics and Gynecology, Yale University School of Medicine

Sara Marder, MD, Assistant Professor of Obstetrics and Gynecology, University of Pennsylvania School of Medicine

Giancarlo Mari, MD, Assistant Professor of Obstetrics and Gynecology, Yale University School of Medicine

Laura McDonald, parent

Sheryl McMahon, parent

Carmen and Justin Murphy, parents

Sherwin B. Nuland, physician and author.

Kunle Odunsi, MD, PhD, MRCOG, Chief Resident, Department of Obstetrics and Gynecology, Yale-New Haven Hospital

Rotimi Odutayo, MD, MRCOG, Department of Obstetrics and Gynecology, Queen's University, Kingston, Ontario, Canada

Tanja Pejovic, MD, PhD, Resident, Department of Obstetrics and Gynecology, Yale-New Haven Hospital

Paolo Rinaudo, MD, Resident, Department of Obstetrics and Gynecology, Yale-New Haven Hospital

Brian and Sue Roquemore, parents

Rene Rylander, parent

Andrea Seigerman, MSW, LCSW, senior clinical social worker, Department of Social Services, Yale-New Haven Hospital

Jacob Tangir, MD, Resident, Department of Obstetrics and Gynecology, Yale-New Haven Hospital

Leena Väisänen, MD, PhD, Faculty of Medicine, University of Oulu, Oulu, Finland

Louise Ward, R.N., MSN, Nurse, Labor and Delivery Suite, Yale-New Haven Hospital, and Codirector, Maternity Bereavement Services, Yale-New Haven Hospital

Ashley Wivel, MD, Yale University School of Medicine

About the Author

MICHAEL R. BERMAN, M.D., FACOG, is Clinical Professor of Obstetrics and Gynecology at Yale University School of Medicine and attending physician, Yale-New Haven Hospital. He is currently the President of the Yale-New Haven Physician Hospital Organization. A graduate of New York Medical College, Dr. Berman is the founder and editor of Hygeia® (www.hygeia.org), a Web site devoted to alleviating the angst of a pregnancy loss or death of a child. He also administers the Hygeia Foundation, Inc., a non-profit organization whose mission is to bring medically indigent and underserved populations, nationally and internationally, interactive information on maternal and child health. Dr. Berman practices obstetrics and gynecology in New Haven and lives in Woodbridge, Connecticut with his wife and two daughters.

www.ingramcontent.com/pod-product-compliance
Lightning Source LLC
Chambersburg PA
CBHW071849270326
41929CB00013B/2156